Healthy Black Hair

Step-by-Step Instructions
for Growing Longer, Stronger Hair

PANACEA PUBLISHING
Bloomfield Hills, MI

Healthy Black Hair

Step-by-Step Instructions for Growing Longer, Stronger Hair

NICOLE ELIZABETH SMITH

PANACEA PUBLISHING
Bloomfield Hills, MI

HEALTHY BLACK HAIR:
STEP-BY-STEP INSTRUCTIONS
FOR GROWING LONGER, STRONGER HAIR

Book design by Michele DeFilippo, 1106 Design, LLC

Edited by Kate von Seeburg

Printed in the United States
on acid-free paper.

If you have any questions or comments
concerning this book, please write:

Panacea Publishing
Book Reader Service
PO Box 395
Bloomfield Hills, MI 48303-0395
www.panaceapublishing.com

ISBN 0-9743432-7-7

Library of Congress Control Number:
2003095332

Publisher's Cataloguing-in-Publication
(Provided by Quality Books, Inc.)

Smith, Nicole Elizabeth.
    Healthy black hair : step-by-step instructions for
growing longer, stronger hair / Nicole Elizabeth Smith.
-- 1st ed.
    p.cm.
    Includes bibliographical references and index.
    LCCN 2003095332
    ISBN 0-9743432-7-7

    1. Hair--Care and hygiene. 2. African American women
--Health and hygiene. 3. Hairdressing of African
Americans. I. Title.

RL91.S65 2003   646.7'24'08996073
                                       QB103-200616

FOR MY SON,
ZACK.

NOTICE

This book is intended as a reference volume only, not as a medical guide or manual for self-treatment. If you suspect that you have a medical problem, please seek competent medical care. This information is designed to help you make informed choices about your hair and health. It is not intended as a substitute for any treatment prescribed by your doctor.

ACKNOWLEDGEMENTS

Thank you Lord, my God, the Father, creator of Heaven and Earth. I am continually awed by your faithfulness, mercy and loving kindness. Thank you for providing the idea, words and resources for me to write this book.

Thanks to my parents, friends and family who supported this crazy idea and provided me with encouragement and support— Mom, Dad, Natalie, Aunt Edna, Aunt Faye and Bruce.

Thank you, Natalie for allowing me to do your hair and rant over its condition; Thank you Mom for watching Zack and supporting me unconditionally; Thank you Dad for providing me free room and board; Thank you Faye for your professional criticism and working under my tight deadline. And Bruce, thanks for supplying me with chocolate contraband, fixing my computers and believing in me.

I appreciate my wonderful and talented book designer Michele DeFilippo so much for keeping my input to a bare minimum; and my editor, Kate von Seeburg, for her sharp eye and valued advice.

Shouts go out to Kendall Dunson for the free legal advice (I owe you lunch) and to John at yogasite.com for the yoga information.

TABLE OF CONTENTS

FOREWORD

Remember the fairy tale about Rapunzel? She was locked in a tower without windows or doors by an evil sorceress. While in captivity, her golden hair grew so long that a prince was able to climb up her hair and rescue her. If Rapunzel was Black, and relaxed her hair, chances are she would still be in that tower!

Why don't more Sisters have long, healthy hair? Are we genetically different from Whites and Asians and simply limited in our hair length? By no means! So it must be something we that are *doing* to our hair that makes it dry and eventually break off. It's our relaxers; chemical straighteners alter our hair physically, leaving it damaged and fragile. That is the reason why we *must* handle our hair with tender loving care.

Who doesn't want beautiful, healthy hair? Growing up, I wanted to be like Rapunzel; when I was a little girl, my hair was long and thick. I wore it in braids, but as I grew older, I begged my mom to let me get a relaxer. I got my first relaxer at age 10 and at first, I was elated! My hair was so soft, silky and manageable. Best of all, I didn't cry every time my mom washed it. But, it didn't last. For years after, I struggled with dry hair and excessive breakage. My hair line was a mess and I had this short patch of hair in the back of my head that simply would not grow. I was shocked to discover that hair grows an average of six inches a year. I didn't

realize that my hair actually *was* growing; the ends just kept breaking off! "Is this it?" I wondered. "Is this simply the fate of Black
women everywhere?" I noticed most of the Black women I knew
had the same short, choppy hair I did, but I refused to give up.
When I got to high school, I pored over Black hair care magazines,
worked with different hair dressers and even spoke to product
manufacturers; however, I could find no common denominator.
They all had their own opinions on what my problem was. I continued struggling with my hair until 1991, when my blow dryer
died, and I splurged and bought the hooded dryer I always
wanted. I discovered how much smoother and straighter my hair
was after a roller set than when I blew it dry. I loved how long the
roller sets lasted and that I could save time in the morning by
wearing rollers at night. And the deep conditioners! When my
hair reached my chin for the first time, I knew I was onto something. I renounced my curling iron, curling brush, portable curling iron, blow dryer, crimping iron, hot comb and hot curlers and
embraced styling my hair without heat. Now, I am able to maintain my hair at home and go to the salon only when I need a touch-
up. Chapter 12 is devoted solely to styling your hair without heat.

As my hair grew I admit I became a bit obsessed. I inspected
every hair that fell out of my head (I still do), took multiple hair
and nail supplements and even made my own hair products but
it seemed my hair had reached its limit. It stopped just above my
shoulders, and nothing I did would make it grow any further. So
finally, frustrated, I simply left it alone. I wore my hair in braids
and in a "helmet" (ponytails covered in protein gel.) I did this
about six months, concentrated on keeping it conditioned, and
bingo! My hair finally broke the shoulder barrier and looked and
felt better than ever. I realized that my hair had gotten "stressed"

and simply needed a Break. Chapter 8 will show you how to put on your "helmet" and achieve the hair length you have always desired. Chapter 9 tells you what supplements you need and which ones you don't.

Armed with a hair care regimen and nutritional plan, I wore my hair long until a couple of years ago, when it mysteriously began to fall out in bunches. The texture changed and it became dry, coarse and brittle again. I tried giving it a Break, but it wouldn't respond to my normal routine. It wasn't the heat, it wasn't my diet, and it wasn't my conditioner. It was my thyroid.

After seeing several doctors, undergoing numerous tests and scans, I was diagnosed with Graves Disease. As it turns out, dry hair and shedding are well known symptoms of thyroid disease; many women claim their thyroid problems were diagnosed by their stylist! Approximately 10 million people in the US have thyroid disease and, unfortunately, too many women go undiagnosed. Could your hair problems be related to thyroid disease? Take the Thyroid Risk Assessment on page 94 to find out.

Getting my body back to normal was easier than getting my hair back together. The medications routinely used to treat thyroid disease only made my situation worse because they can cause hair loss as well. The doctors knew how to fix my thyroid, but they couldn't (or wouldn't) fix my hair. My hair loss became so severe that I eventually purchased a wig. It was then that I realized that healthy hair comes from the inside; all of the cosmetics in the world can only enhance what must already exist. Our hair is a barometer of our internal state. If we are feeling tired, sick or depressed, it will show up in our hair. With this new outlook, I conducted my own research on the thyroid gland, the hormones it produces and thyroid medications. What I discovered helped me get my hair healthy again. You can learn what I discovered in Chapter 11, "Your Thyroid and Your Hair."

So many Black women suffer needlessly with breakage, dandruff and dull, dry hair. When my sister complained that she just didn't have the "knack" for styling her hair like I do, I realized it was time to share what I have learned. There are no expensive products to buy, no "natural" ways to straighten your hair and no magic pills; just straightforward, proven techniques to rejuvenate your hair and improve its growth. I hope you will find this information complete, concise and easy to follow.

I would love to hear from you! Email your testimonials, questions and comments to Nicole@hbhonline.com.

Good luck!

*"…if a woman has long hair,
it is a glory to her:
for her hair is given her
for a covering."*
— 1 Corinthians 11:15

1

INTRODUCTION

Congratulations! You are on your way to having the long, luxurious hair you've always dreamed of. Regardless of what texture your hair is your hair can be healthier and three inches longer in just six months. Through the 5 Principles of Healthy Hair you will learn how to maintain your hair at home and how to give your hair a Break for outstanding growth. The foundation of this program is styling your hair without heat. Sound impossible? I have been doing it for years and included step by-step instructions to help you create five different hair-styles.

The 5 Principles of Healthy Hair are:

1. **Eat** a healthy diet and take supplements to give your hair the nutrients it needs to grow.

2. **Stimulate your hair and scalp**. Good circulation helps bring nutrients and oxygen to your hair and scalp.

3. **Prevent** damage by avoiding heat, over-processing and harsh styling.

4. **Protect** your hair, especially the ends, from sun damage, chemicals and fabrics.

5. **Treat** hair and scalp disorders to relieve dandruff and stop hair loss.

WHO IS THIS BOOK FOR?

This book is for any woman who regularly relaxes her hair. You may be stuck in the same cycle of hair breakage that I was and are frustrated because it seems as if your hair has been the same length forever. Or, you may not be concerned about how long your hair is but just want it to be healthy. It is possible! Regardless of what texture your hair is (fine, thin, coarse or just plain nappy) you can have long, healthy hair. Think of this as a fitness program for your hair, and like getting in shape, it will take time, effort and consistency.

Many women grow their hair out natural thinking that will make their hair easier to manage. They soon find out that natural hair takes longer to care for and is more expensive to maintain. Relaxers were created to make caring for our hair easier, not to emulate another race. If you have trouble finding the time to maintain your hair, check out some time saving tips on page 41.

LET'S GET REAL

However, some hair is so soft, it can't take a perm. This kind of hair will break off no matter how well you treat it. My friend Nikkia's hair is nappy like mine, but it is baby-fine and the natural color is light brown. No matter what Nikkia did, her hair would not grow to chin length, so one day she went to a barber shop and got a fade! Cut it all off; she was bold, but she was right.

That was three years ago and her hair has since grown past her shoulders. She wears it in twists and braids and the styles suit her. She did what was best for her. You have to figure out what is best for you.

Genetics means as much as the condition your hair is in (healthy, dry or damaged). Does your hair respond well to a perm or does is it continually break? Every Black woman's hair texture is different but a perm should make it lighter and easier to manage. My sister's hair is thicker than mine but we both take perms well. Is your hair shinier and more manageable after a perm? If the answer is yes, and you want to continue to straighten it, read on.

2

YOUR CROWNING GLORY

Before we get into styling, let's start with the fundamentals.

BASIC HAIR STRUCTURE

Your hair has two separate parts: the **root** and the **shaft**.

Root

The root is the part of the hair located just under the skin surface. The **hair follicle** houses the entire hair root. The **papilla** is where all of the action takes place; it is a rich blood and nerve supply that nourishes the hair shaft and produces hair cells. The bulb is a white sack located on the lower part of the hair that covers the papilla. Caucasian hair follicles point straight up; however, in Black hair the hair follicle has a "c" shape, forcing the hair to grow up in a corkscrew. This unique shape is the reason our hair is has a tendency to be dry and is so easily damaged. Caucasian hair can get greasy because it is straight (oil just slides down the hair shaft) but our curls prevent oil from being distributed throughout our hair.

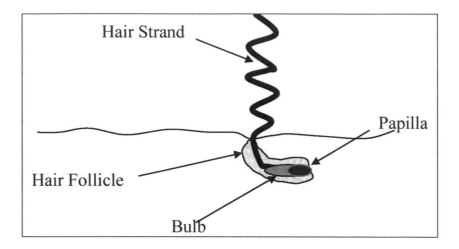

Shaft

The hair shaft is what is grows out of the hair follicle and is what we consider to be hair. It has three parts; the **cuticle, cortex** and **medulla**. Hair is made of dead **keratin** (protein) cells that are pushed up through the scalp at an average rate of about one-half inch per month for six inches of hair growth each year. Because hair is dead, once it is damaged, it cannot be repaired. Many products claim to repair hair, but all they do is temporarily "glue" your hair back together. Therefore, your hair must be treated gently, especially while styling, and the damaged hair, cut off.

The outer layer of your hair shaft is called the cuticle, which holds your hair together. The cells or scales that make up the cuticle layer overlap similarly to the scales on a fish or the shingles on a roof. This is your hair's armor; it protects the heart, or the cortex, the layer beneath the cuticle. It is made of long, molecular chains of amino acids (protein) and is the largest section of your hair. Chemical straighteners must penetrate through the cuticle to access the cortex, where shape and color changes take place.

Melanin in the cortex determines what color your hair will be. Permanent hair colors deposit or remove color from the cortex to make your hair appear lighter or darker. The medulla is the center most part of the hair shaft. It gives the hair stiffness and may be fragmented. It is sometimes even absent, resulting in extremely soft, limp hair.

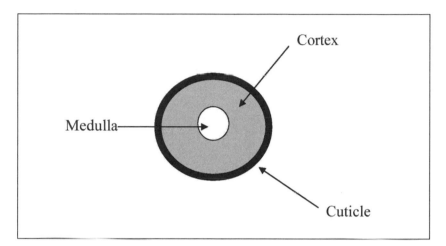

In healthy hair, the cuticle scales lay flat, which traps moisture and reflects light, making the hair look shiny. Chemicals, heat and harsh styling (fine tooth combs, boar bristles brushes, back combing or ratting hair) can damage and even break the cuticle scales, making your hair look dull and feel rough.

Ideally, your hair's composition is about 90% protein and 10% water. Yes, water! Water *is* moisture, so when your hair becomes dry, it needs water, not oil or grease as we have been taught to believe. Oil can, however, help keep your hair supple, if it is the right kind. Natural oils such as olive or jojoba oil can penetrate the cuticle layer; others (petroleum-based), cannot. Since hair cannot soak up petroleum-based hair greases, guess what? It sits on the hair and scalp, weighs hair down, and makes it look dirty.

Since your hair needs moisture, and water is moisture, this means we need to wash and condition our hair frequently. It is for this reason that I recommend that you wash and deep condition your hair twice a week or when your hair starts to feel dry. This is contrary to another myth we grew up with, that washing your hair dries it out. Frequent washing helps your hair by replenishing moisture and removing product build-up. Shampoos, hair sprays and gel leave a film on your hair known as product build-up. This build-up covers your hair shaft and can prevent your hair from absorbing moisture. Regular washing can remove those products and prevent that from happening.

POROSITY

In hair care, porosity is your hair's ability to absorb moisture and chemicals. Think of your hair as a sponge, and just like a sponge it can soak up and hold a certain amount of water and natural oil. Healthy hair has good porosity. The cuticle layer is raised over the cortex allowing conditioner, oil and water to be absorbed into the hair shaft, then held in by the cuticle scales. Over-processed or damaged hair has poor porosity. This kind of hair is unable to retain moisture because there is no room for it between the layers and the damaged cuticle scales are unable to hold the moisture in. After porosity is degraded, there is no way to restore it.

THE GROWTH PROCESS

There are three distinct stages in the hair growth cycle: **anagen**, **catagen** and **telogen**. However, the life length and growth cycle of each hair varies. For example, your hair grows best in the summer, in warm climates and between the ages of 18–35.

Anagen, or the growing stage, can last from a few months to several years, during which the length, texture and thickness of your hair are determined. Normally, 80%–90% of your hair follicles are in the anagen stage. Anagen phases differ from person to person. In some people, anagen may be several years; in others, just a few.

Catagen, the resting or holding phase, should last a few weeks. During this phase, your hair is attached to the scalp but no growth takes place. This allows the hair bulb to slowly separate from the follicle base, readying itself for removal. Approximately 1% of your hair follicles will be in the catagen phase simultaneously.

Telogen, the re-growth phase, can last for three or four months. This is the renewal period for the hair follicle. The hair follicle will remain dormant (asleep) until going into a new anagen phase, giving birth to a new hair strand. This new strand will push up and out, causing the old one to be shed. Hair that is shed in this stage will leave the scalp intact with a white bulb attached to the end. We can lose 75–100 hairs per day due to this process. Approximately 10% to 15% of your scalp follicles are in telogen simultaneously.

WHAT CAN GO WRONG?

Diffuse hair loss (telogen effluvium) occurs when a large number of hair follicles enter the telogen phase prematurely and abruptly. This can occur as a result of thyroid disease (Chapter 11), medication (read your prescription insert for a list of side effects) and even stress.

Alopecia areata is characterized by bald spots, which can occur anywhere on the head, especially around the hairline. It is an autoimmune skin disorder that causes severe hair loss. Alopecia can also be caused by an under-active thyroid (hypothyroidism). Autoimmune diseases are when the body's own immune system (white blood cells) attacks itself. In this case, white blood cells attack the hair follicles, causing them to shut down. Alopecia usually starts out slowly, with one small bald patch, and continues to spread. Sometimes, this hair loss can be reversed. If you are experiencing bald spots, consult a dermatologist.

Postpartum alopecia is hair loss that occurs after childbirth. During pregnancy, the body's elevated estrogen level causes our hair to "freeze" in the growth phase. Hair that would normally have shed (75–100 per day) continues to grow or hold steady. After childbirth, however, the estrogen levels fall and so does your hair. Beginning in the third or fourth month postpartum, the hair may shed at an alarming rate. This is normal and should decrease by the sixth month postpartum. If your hair loss continues, talk with your doctor.

Aging affects our hair in different ways. Over the years, hair texture can change and the number of follicles capable of growing hair declines. As we age the period of anagen (growth) shortens, which leads to hair thinning. This process begins in the mid 30's and increases as we get older. The decline is especially noticeable on the top of the head and around the temple. If you are experiencing natural, age-related hair loss, you can try using minoxidil to re-grow your hair or talk with your doctor about other treatment options.

pH

You may have heard people talking about **pH** levels in shampoos and conditioners. pH stands for potential hydrogen. It is a measure of alkalinity and acidity on a scale of 1–14. A number 7 is neutral; water has a pH level of 7. Any number above 7 is considered alkaline; below 7, acidic.

The normal pH level of your hair is between 4.5 and 5.5. Lye perms have a pH level of 12–14 and no-lye perms are 10–12, so after being permed your hair may be left with a higher pH level. To help stabilize hair pH levels, always choose a shampoo with pH level between 4.5 and 5.5. Most shampoos will fall into this category; but some medicinal shampoos (i.e. dandruff shampoos) are much higher.

YOUR HEALTHY HAIR DIARY

To truly give your hair the attention it needs, you should use and maintain a Healthy Hair Diary. Use your Healthy Hair Diary to fill out the tests in Chapters 3 and 4, note how hair feels on your start date and track its progress. If you really want to motivate yourself, measure your hair from the scalp to the ends on your start date, then measure after every perm to track your growth.

Your hair diary is a great way to remember which relaxer brands have been used on your hair, what shampoos and conditioners give you the best results and when you received your last perm and trim. I don't know about you, but I forget the date of my perms and refer to my diary often! Utilize this diary to note changes in your hair so you can see what vitamins and/or products work best on your hair and which ones don't make a difference. You can purchase your Healthy Hair Diary at your local bookstore.

SUMMARY

• Normal hair loss is 75–100 hairs a day

• The hair shaft has three layers, the cuticle (outer), the cortex (middle) and medulla (core)

• Hair grows in three stages, anagen (growth), catagen and telogen (re-growth)

• Normal hair pH level is between 4.5 and 5.5

NOTES:

_____

_____

_____

_____

_____

_____

_____

_____

_____

3

YOUR SCALP

Unfortunately, we have made caring for our scalp more difficult than it has to be. All your scalp needs to be happy is to be kept clean and stimulated.

Tradition gives us many unhealthy habits. Growing up, I would grease my scalp, scratch it with a fine tooth comb and pour Seabreeze® on it thinking I was curing dandruff. If that was the case, why did it persist? Visible scales or build-up on the scalp is not normal and usually indicates a scalp disorder. These symptoms should not be accepted or ignored. Although most disorders do not cause permanent hair loss, they should be treated before they lead to hair shedding or a stunted hair follicle. For instance, as hair grows out of the follicle it can get stuck in the scales, then be pulled out by the root when the scale is removed (through picking or scratching). Also, dandruff provides resistance to your hair follicle, making it more difficult for your hair to grow. If your hair is unable to grow out of the hair follicle, it (your hair follicle) will shut down. Thankfully, this is usually temporary, and the follicle will move into the anagen phase once the problem is treated.

COMPOSITION

Your scalp is part of the body's largest organ, the skin. The skin on your scalp is thicker than the skin on your body and has more hair follicles (around 250,000). About 100,000 of those follicles are active (anagen) at one time. Your scalp has two main parts; the dermis and the **epidermis**.

The epidermis is the top layer of your skin, resting on top of the dermis. The dermis, or the lower layer, is composed of connective tissue, blood vessels, hair follicles and sebaceous glands. The sebaceous glands secrete sebum, oil which lubricates your hair and scalp. Because your scalp creates its own oil, you do not need to grease your scalp. When used on your scalp, petroleum-based hair grease can clog your pores, attract dirt and prevent healing oxygen from reaching your scalp. A healthy scalp should be loose (able to move), thick and smooth, without any visible redness or rashes.

SCALP DISORDERS

The most common scalp disorder is **dandruff,** or **pityriasis capitis simplex.** However, dandruff is a term we mistakenly use to describe a variety of symptoms including itching, flaking or dry scalp. What we think is dandruff may actually be **dermatitis** or **scalp psoriasis.**

An itchy scalp is not always caused by dandruff. If you are primarily experiencing scalp itch without flakes, stress could be the cause. Chill out! To alleviate the symptoms, learn stress management techniques, pray actively, practice yoga exercises or take a vacation.

In your Healthy Hair Diary, mark your answers to the test on the following pages to help determine the health of your scalp.

SCALP HEALTH ASSESSMENT

1. **Does your scalp itch?**
   a. Yes
   b. No
   c. Sometimes

2. **If yes, does it itch after a shampoo or does it take a few days to reoccur?**
   a. After shampoo
   b. After a few days

3. **Do you see flakes or scales on your scalp? If yes, are the flakes:**
   a. Large and greasy, gray in color
   b. Small and round, white in color
   c. Silver, powdery scales

4. **Does the majority of your flaking occur on the top (center) of your head?**
   a. Yes
   b. No

5. **Do you sometimes see dark brown flakes, flakes with a red dot or scabs?**
   a. Yes
   b. No

6. **Does anything (shampoo, oil or medication) help or stop the itch?**
   a. Yes
   b. No

(continued on next page)

7. Are the scales accompanied with redness or greasy scales
on your face, eyebrows or eyelashes?
a. Yes
b. No

8. Do you have psoriasis on your body?
a. Yes
b. No

Check your answers on page 115. Use this as a guide to increase your awareness and help pinpoint any problems you may have. This is not to be considered a diagnosis. If your scalp problems persist, please seek professional medical advice.

DANDRUFF

Your skin continually sheds itself every 24 days, including the skin on your scalp. That's what dandruff is; dead skin cells being shed as part of your body's normal renewal and growth process. This type of dandruff is characterized by dry, white flakes and can be managed by washing your hair twice a week and exfoliating your scalp.

Problems occur, however, when your scalp begins to shed skin cells at an excessive rate, called **pityriasis steatoides**. In some cases, the skin cells are still alive! This can occur for any number of reasons including the presence of the fungus **pityrosporum ovale**. This kind of dandruff is contagious, will smell bad and looks like large, greasy clumps of scales. Because this and other types of dandruff are considered contagious, do not use other people's combs or brushes.

Symptoms

• Large, greasy clumps of flakes (abnormal dandruff)

• Dry, white flakes (normal dandruff)

• White or gray patches of scales, usually located on the top of the head (both)

• Itching (both)

Treatment

There are several treatments available for controlling both types of dandruff. Shampoos that contain coal tar, salicylic acid, sulfur or selenium sulfide such as Nizoral® and Neutrogena T-gel® can help remove flakes and relieve itching. However, use them sparingly. Overuse can dry your hair.

To control dandruff follow these steps:

1. **Supplement your diet with Essential Fatty Acids.** See page 81 for more information.

2. **Disinfect all of your combs and plastic brushes** in a sanitizing solution of 1 cup bleach to 4 cups water. Scrub them well and let them soak for at least 10 minutes. Boil metal hair clips in hot water and/or bleach solution for 10–15 minutes.

3. **Wash your hair with a dandruff shampoo.** For best results, put the shampoo on your scalp, not your hair. Lather, rinse and lather again, then place a plastic cap on your head and let the shampoo sit for 5–10 minutes. Rinse and follow with a deep conditioner. Style as usual. The next time you shampoo return to using your regular shampoo; however, continue to disinfect

your combs and brushes at every shampoo (until your dandruff clears up.) If your hair is very dry, try washing your hair first with a moisturizing shampoo then washing with the dandruff shampoo. Allow it sit on your scalp for up to 5 minutes.

4. **Massage your scalp.** To help remove and relieve dandruff, massage oil infused with an essential oil like rosemary or lavender onto your scalp. Tea tree oil can be applied directly to your scalp (use sparingly) to relieve itching.

5. **Apply hot oil treatments.** They condition your hair as well as your scalp, and when performed prior to shampoo, help remove dandruff.

6. **Never "scratch" or "lift" your dandruff** with a comb; doing so may cause irritation or infection and might make your condition worse. Instead, gently exfoliate your scalp during your shampoo.

Exfoliation is the process of removing dead skin cells (dandruff) from your scalp, revealing healthy, new skin. To exfoliate your scalp, use a scalp brush (see page 56). After working your shampoo into a lather, place your scalp massager on your scalp and move it back and forth using small, short strokes. Do not try to rake the brush through your hair, but work it back and forth in one spot, and then place it in another area. Work your way around your head, then rinse. Keep your massager clean by rinsing it out then drying it with the bristles down.

DERMATITIS

Dermatitis is a skin disorder characterized by dryness and itching that does not respond to moisture. Studies have shown that continued exposure to sodium hydroxide (lye) can cause dermatitis.[1]

Symptoms

• Dry Scalp

• Tiny white flakes (may look like dry skin)

• Persistent itching

• Occasional redness

If this describes the symptoms you are experiencing and your situation does not respond to the treatment for dandruff, please see a dermatologist for treatment options.

SCALP PSORIASIS

Normally, it takes about a month for new skin cells to move from the lower layers to the surface. In psoriasis, it takes only a few days, resulting in a build-up of dead skin cells and thick scales. Psoriasis is a very common condition, affecting approximately three million Americans, but it is not contagious. Psoriasis is genetic and related to an inflammatory response in which the immune system mistakenly targets the body's own cells. It can appear very suddenly and may occur repeatedly. The disorder can affect people of any age, but it most commonly begins between the ages of 15 and 35.

Symptoms

* Lesions on the scalp

* Psoriasis on other parts of the body

* Patches of silver scales on the scalp that start small and then grow larger

* May be accompanied by redness

If you are exhibiting any of the symptoms of scalp psoriasis or you have psoriasis on other parts of your body, please seek professional medical advice. Treatments for scalp psoriasis include medicated shampoos, steroids, topical medications and ultraviolet (UV) light.

NOTES:

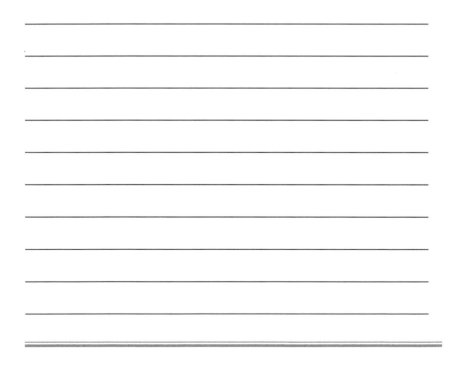

4

WHAT ARE YOU WORKIN' WITH?

Before we go any further, let's determine what kind of hair you have. By what kind, I mean the condition, not the so-called "grade."

In your hair diary, write your answers to the questions on the following pages to help determine the current condition of your hair. Once we know what we're working with, we can formulate an appropriate hair care regimen.

HAIR TYPE TEST

1. Collect a few strands of your hair. Pull a strand. Did it stretch before breaking?
   a. Yes
   b. No

2. Take a look at the strands you collected. Do they have a white bulb at the end?
   a. Yes
   b. No

(continued on next page)

3. Is your hair dull or shiny?
 a. Dull
 b. Shiny

4. Do you take a daily multi–vitamin?
 a. Yes
 b. No

5. Do you diet frequently?
 a. Yes
 b. No

6. Do you take thyroid medication?
 a. Yes
 b. No

7. Is your hair breaking (short hair strands)?
 a. Yes
 b. No

8. Is your hair shedding (long hair strands)?
 a. Yes
 b. No

9. Does your hair hold a curl well?
 a. Yes
 b. No

10. How many times a week do you use heat to style your hair?
 a. 0
 b. 1–2
 c. 3–5
 d. 6–7

11. Do you blow dry your hair?

    a. Yes

    b. No

    c. Sometimes

Use the answer key on page 116 to find out your score.

Healthy: 0–8 points

Congratulations on taking such great care of your hair! Hair that is healthy is sexy and beautiful! Whether you maintain your hair yourself or have a great hairdresser, you should be proud. Now, let's keep that hair, shall we?

Characteristics of Healthy Hair

• Smooth texture and feel

• Shiny

• Hair loss is 75–100 strands per day

• Hair loss consists of entire hair strands (contains bulb)

• Holds curl well

• Relatively easy to comb while wet

• Good elasticity (hair strand stretches when pulled)

• Healthy scalp

• No breakage

• Minimal split ends

Cause and Effect

Healthy hair is our goal. In hair that is in good condition, the outer layer (cuticle) is smooth which helps the hair retain moisture. In your hair diary make a detailed list of things are you doing to keep you hair in such good condition. Examples include: deep conditioning, frequent hair trims and using a wide tooth comb.

Check your reasons against the list of Do's and Don'ts on page 117. Make a vow to stop doing anything on the Don'ts list and give some of the Do's a try.

Your Hair Regimen:

- Wash your hair twice weekly using a protein or moisturizing shampoo

- Deep condition at least once a week (with heat)

- Limit the use of heat (curling irons, etc.) to once a week or emergencies

- Daily multi-vitamins

- Hair trims twice a year

- Regular perms every 7–9 weeks

- Take a Break at least once a year for an entire perm cycle

- Stimulate your scalp regularly

Be careful not to get complacent or lazy with your hair care. Your hair is healthy now, but that does not mean it can take some abuse. Flip to Chapter 7 to learn how to maintain your hair and watch it grow!

Stressed (Dry): 10–18 points

Kinky hair can easily become dry or stressed from the heat and chemicals we use in styling. You are in the danger zone! Hair that is in the stressed category is on its way to becoming damaged. On the other hand, if you make some hair care changes now, your hair can become healthy!

Characteristics of Stressed Hair

• Hair loss is 75–100+ per day

• Hair is dry to the touch but responds well to moisture

• May have some scalp problems

• Dull appearance

• Itchy scalp

• Loses curl easily

• May be frizzy

• Hair has poor elasticity (does not stretch before breaking)

• Breakage (hair strands are short)

• Split ends

Cause and Effect

The scales on the outer layer of your hair shaft are not smooth. Some may even be missing which upsets your hair's moisture balance and makes it dry. How did your hair become dry? In your hair diary make a detailed list of reasons why you believe your hair is "stressed." Some examples include the daily use of a curling iron, blow-drying or use of permanent hair color.

Read the list of Do's and Don'ts on page 117. Are you a repeat offender? Are you addicted to your blow dryer or is your diet simply lacking in nutrients? Whatever the reasons, now that you are aware of what you are doing wrong, you can make a conscious decision to change. Remember: Small changes in the way you care for your can make the difference between hair that is four inches long, and hair that is 18 inches long!

Your Hair Regimen

• Begin your regimen with a Break for at least six weeks

• Continue to take a Break at least once a year for 6–8 weeks

• Wash twice weekly with a protein shampoo

• Use a protein treatment immediately to stop breakage

• Deep condition twice a week (preferably with heat)

• No-heat styling

• Daily multi-vitamins

• Hair trims 2–3 times a year

• Regular perms every 7–9 weeks

• Increase scalp circulation

Your healthy hair regimen will be detailed Chapter 7. Also, your hair needs to take a Break. For more information see Chapter 8.

Damaged: 19 + points

Damaged hair, while the most challenging to work with, is also the most rewarding. You have the potential for greatness! Once you figure out how, when and why your hair is damaged, you can learn from your mistakes and not repeat them. In damaged hair the cuticle scales are raised, uneven or completely destroyed, resulting in hair that is dry, brittle and easily tangled, especially when wet. Unlike your body, your hair does not have the ability to repair itself. Once the hair is damaged, no product in the world can repair it permanently.

Characteristics of Damaged Hair

• Dull

• Dry

• Coarse

• Frequent use of oil does not help retain moisture and/or the effects do not last long

• Tangles easily, difficult to comb while wet

• Frizzy

• Breakage is severe in spots

• Visible split ends

• Scalp may be unhealthy

• May have excessive dandruff

Cause and Effect

How did your hair become damaged? Make a detailed list of reasons how your hair became damaged (daily use of a curling iron, permanent hair color plus relaxer, etc.). If you don't know, check the list of Don'ts on page 119. You may be surprised to see a lot of things you are doing! Make a vow to stop doing the Don'ts and things you listed above then incorporate the Do's into your daily routine. If you start now, your hair can be six inches longer this time next year!

Your Hair Regimen

• Start with a good trim or haircut

• Use a protein treatment immediately to stop breakage

• Follow with an extended Break, at least six weeks (preferably 12)

• After your Break, wash your hair twice weekly with a protein shampoo

• Bi-weekly deep conditioner (preferably with heat)

• No-heat styling

• Regular perms every 7–9 weeks

• No chemicals other than relaxers, including semi-permanent colors

• Hair trims 2–3 times per year

Keep in mind that damaged hair can be a vicious cycle. Chapter 7 will show you the right way to care for your hair. But first, give your hair an extended Break (Chapter 8) for up to 12 weeks to really revive your locks. You can do it!

The next chapter will help you choose the right product for your hair type. If your hair is dry or damaged, don't feel bad. It doesn't matter where you begin; it matters where you end up!

NOTES:

5

GATHER YOUR SUPPLIES

We have some shopping to do! In this chapter, you will learn about the products you need and how to choose them. There's no need to spend a bundle; it is possible to spend as little as $20 for your shampoo, conditioner and styling aids.

Got your pen and pencil ready? Here is the list of items you will need:

- Shampoo

- Plastic caps

- Deep moisturizing conditioner

- Protein Treatment

- Instant conditioner

- Wide tooth comb

- Fine tooth comb

- Hair gloss (shine)

- Healthy Hair Diary

- Leave-in conditioner

- Light hair oil

- Heavy hair oil

- Setting lotion

- Protein gel

- Rollers and clips

- Night-time head wrap

SHAMPOO

All hair types will benefit from a strengthening protein shampoo. Protein shampoos coat your hair shaft with protein (filling in the gaps) to make it stronger. The pH level, if listed, should be between 4.5 and 5.5. However, if your hair is already healthy, you may choose to use a moisturizing shampoo if a protein shampoo makes your hair feel coarse. When choosing your shampoo, check the label. Look for proteins and mild **surfactants** (cleansing agents) in the list of ingredients. Gentle surfactants or cleansing agents include **sodium laureth sulfate, ammonium laureth sulfate** and **ammonium laurel sulfate**. There are numerous proteins that may be included; keratin, collagen, **amino acids** or **hydrolyzed wheat proteins** are just a few.

Recommendations:

- Botanoil® by Nexxus

- Keracare® Hydrating/Detangling Shampoo

• Suave® Professionals Humectant Shampoo

• Mane and Tale® (protein) Shampoo

• Aphoghee® Shampoo for Damaged Hair (protein)

Tip: Keep a bottle of Cream of Nature on hand for emergencies. Use it after removing braids or just before a perm to make your hair easier to detangle.

PLASTIC CAP

You can never have too many of these. You can use them for deep conditioning, hot oil treatments and as shower caps. Buy them in bulk so you always have one on hand.

DEEP MOISTURIZING CONDITIONER

Deep conditioners can be applied with or without heat and work in 10–35 minutes. This is the most critical product in your regimen, so choose wisely. Always check the list of ingredients for oils (coconut, wheat germ, etc.), **humectants** and **finishing agents.** Humectants attract moisture to the hair like a magnet and include **glycerin, propylene glycol** and **sorbitol.** Finishing agents help stick the hair back together, detangle and impart shine. **Dimethicone, mineral oil** and **cymethicone** are excellent finishing agents.

Tip: If you don't have a lot of money to spend, purchase an inexpensive protein shampoo, but buy a good conditioner.

Recommendations:

• Terax® Crema

• Motions® at home moisture plus conditioner

• Keracare Humecto®

PROTEIN TREATMENT

This product will be used once in a perm cycle, usually in the week after you get your perm. The purpose of a protein treatment is to help strengthen your hair by filling in the damaged cuticle layer. We learned in Chapter 2 that once hair is damaged, it cannot be repaired. However, damaged hair strands have "dents" that can be temporarily filled and smoothed over with this type of protein product. These products can stop breakage immediately and the effects will last for several weeks. You will be amazed at the results! Due to their infrequent use, one bottle may last you 6–12 months.

Recommendations:

• For damaged hair: Aphogee® Treatment for Damaged Hair and Balancing Moisturizer (the two go together)

• For healthy hair only: Nexxus Emergencee®

• For all hair types: Mizani Kerafuse® and Moisturefuse® Protein Treatment (the two go together). This is a salon treatment and prices vary. If you do use this at home, make sure your mixture is 1 part Kerafuse® to 3 (1:3) parts Moisturefuse®.

INSTANT CONDITIONER

I am one of those people who believe you just can't condition your hair too much. I always follow my deep conditioner with an instant conditioner. An instant conditioner should make your hair feel soft and tangle free. It is also useful on those days when you simply do not have time to deep condition your hair. These conditioners work in 1–5 minutes.

Recommendations:

• Humectress® by Nexxus

• Keraphix® by Nexxus

• Mane and Tale® Conditioner

• Suave® Professionals Humectant Conditioner

HOODED DRYER

Consider this an investment. Buy a standard hooded dryer with multiple temperature settings. Hooded dryers are versatile, portable and inexpensive (about $35). Some even have radios that play under the hood to keep you from getting bored. Grab a book, get comfortable!

WIDE TOOTH COMB

A wide tooth comb will be your standard styling tool. Use it for the majority of your hairstyling, especially when your hair is wet. Wide tooth combs can part, detangle and section your hair with ease.

FINE TOOTH COMB

Choose a sturdy fine tooth comb with coated teeth. A rat tail is an added plus for making parts and dividing hair. Use your fine tooth comb sparingly and only after detangling with a wide tooth comb. Fine tooth combs can do a lot of damage to both wet and dry hair; the teeth can snag cuticles scales or tear tangled hair out.

GLOSS (SHINE)

I love this stuff! This ultra-light product helps detangle wet hair by providing a slippery surface for your comb to slide through. It also makes your hair glossy once it dries. It can be used on wet and dry hair, will not leave your hair greasy looking and will lock in moisture. There are several good products on the market and prices vary widely. **Be sure to purchase the bottle and not a spray.** Look for **silicone** and **dimethicone** as the major ingredients.

Recommendations

- Proclaim® Glossing polish

- Biosilk® (contains silk proteins)

LEAVE-IN CONDITIONER

Leave-in conditioners help keep your hair moisturized in between shampoos. They should not make your hair feel waxy or sticky. Choose a leave-in conditioner with sunscreen like **octyl methoxycinnamate** to help protect your hair from the sun. Look for **panthenol** (B vitamin), humecants and proteins in the list of ingredients.

Recommendations:

• Infusion®

• Headdress by Nexxus®

• Mane and Tale® conditioner (can also be used as a leave-in)

SCALP BRUSH

This tool looks like a suction cup with plastic "bristles." There are several different kinds to choose from. Choose the massager with the sturdiest bristles that are about ¼" inch apart. Stay away from anything that looks too much like a brush. Scalp massagers help exfoliate dead skin cells off your scalp, remove dandruff and increase circulation. The cost is nominal, about 75 cents each.

LIGHT HAIR OIL

This will be used every day to help moisturize your hair, primarily the ends, but can also be used in small amounts on your scalp. Natural oil, which is absorbed better, can also be used as the base of your massage oil. They are available at any health food store.

Recommendations:

• Jojoba Oil

• Almond oil

• Olive oil

• Wheat germ oil

HEAVY HAIR OIL

These products may contain petroleum. Why is this OK when we know our hair and scalp cannot absorb petroleum? That's the point! We want to create a *physical* barrier between your hair and your cosmetics, especially your facial cleanser. If the grease were absorbed, it would defeat the purpose. It is not for use on the scalp, but feel free to use it on the ends of your hair. Apply it to your hairline morning and night.

Recommendations:

• Royal Crown®

PROTEIN HAIR GEL

Any kind will do, but make sure it is a true protein gel by looking for protein in the list of ingredients. Why use protein gel but not styling gel? You should be sensing a pattern here. The protein in the gel will help to strengthen your hair and the gel itself will dry hard, physically protecting the hair from sun, wind and pollution. Hair sprays, mousse and non-protein styling gels contain alcohols which can dry your hair.

SETTING LOTION

Setting lotion will be used in all your healthy hair styles. It can be used undiluted for hard, crispy curls or diluted with water for loose, bouncy waves. A 1 part setting lotion to 1 part water (1:1, equal amounts) is a great solution for roller sets. For loose curls and wraps, use a 1 part setting lotion to 4 part water solution (1:4). Buy a plastic spray bottle for easy measuring, storage and application.

Recommendations:

• Lottabody® Texturizing Setting Lotion

• Wrap 'n Tap®

ROLLERS AND CLIPS

Most beauty supply stores sell roller starter kits that contain a variety of sizes. For roller sets, choose magnetic rollers without the snap-on cover (covers leave dents) and avoid sponge or cloth rollers. However, for overnight use, rollers with snap-on covers can come in handy. Depending on the length of your hair, you will need 12–36 rollers plus the same number of clips. Bobby pins with coated ends can also be used. Choose your roller size based on the length of your hair and the results desired.

• ¼ inch rollers   Short hair or tight curls in medium to long hair

• ½ inch rollers   Short and medium hair curls, spiral curls for long hair

• 1 inch rollers   Loose curls for medium to long hair

• 1½ inch rollers   Waves and body for long hair

NIGHT-TIME HAIR WRAP

You need a scarf or bonnet to protect your hair's *style* and a satin pillowcase to protect your *hair*. Purchase a large, satin bonnet to cover rollers and satin scarf or do rag to tie up wraps. If you lose your scarf at night like I do, a satin pillowcase is a great backup. Beware of cotton pillowcases! Cotton robs your hair of moisture and the friction caused from tossing and turning can dry, tangle or even break your hair.

STORING YOUR SUPPLIES

Find a convenient spot to store your supplies and keep them handy. Here are some helpful hints:

• Install an étagère above your toilet for added storage space.

• Store your rollers and clips separately to speed up a roller set.

• Stow your rollers in a plastic bin with a drawer or snap-on cover.

• Keep ponytail holders and clips in a small plastic container (empty perm container) with a lid or in an accessories caddy.

• Install a shower caddy for quick access to your shampoo and conditioner.

• Store homemade solutions in inexpensive plastic applicator bottles.

MAKING TIME FOR YOUR HAIR

Healthy hair care takes time. If you don't have time to care for your hair, that probably means you need to! Expect to spend about 6–7 hours a week on your hair. This includes twice weekly hair washing and dryer time. Sound outrageous? How much time do you spend getting your hair done at the salon?

I used to spend four hours twice a week on my hair. However, after I had my son, all of that went out the window. I still wash my hair twice a week, or every four days, but now I save time by air-drying my hair or doing housework with my conditioner on. Don't skip hair washing due to lack of time. As mothers and wives, we dictate the mood of the household. If you don't look good, you don't feel good, and everyone in the house will suffer. Set aside some beauty time for yourself: relax and enjoy it. You're worth it!

Here are some time saving tips:

- Wash your hair before going to bed or while your kids are asleep.

- Air-dry your hair overnight.

- Apply deep conditioner then walk the treadmill or do house work. Raising your body temperature will help the conditioner penetrate.

- Give yourself a facial or paint your toenails while deep conditioning your hair.

- Take a Break during busy times or get braids for a perm cycle.

- Let your hair grow out. Contrary to popular belief, longer hair does not take longer to style. With long hair, you have more hairstyles to choose from, including ponytails and up-do's.

- Fake it. Keep a **drawstring ponytail** or clip-on bun on hand for emergencies.

SUMMARY

The cosmetics industry is booming and it seems new products are added every day. How do you know which one is right for your hair? **When shopping for products, remember the following rules:**

1. **Read the ingredients.** Familiarize yourself with cosmetic ingredients and read the labels. Remember, products are listed in the order of quantity. The first product listed is in the largest amount.

2. **Buy a trusted name.** Purchase products used in your salon such as Mizani,® Nexxus® and Keracare.® If you buy products from established manufacturers, most of them will stand by their product. If you are not satisfied, simply return them for a full refund.

3. **Get a recommendation.** Ask a friend, family member or your hair stylist for recommendations.

4. **You get what you pay for.** There are some great buys out there, such as Suave's® Professional line, but keep in mind that these products can only imitate the originals.

5. **Be smart.** Product manufacturers are in business to sell products and make money. Some of them will make outrageous claims to hook you. If it sounds too good to be true, it usually is.

6. **Buy shampoo and conditioner** from the same product line. Products from the same product family contain similar ingredients that complement each other.

7. **Natural isn't always better.** Many products make claims that their "natural" product is better for your hair. Natural and botanical products are great, but many of these products don't have enough of the natural ingredients in them to truly make a difference. Be a savvy consumer and read the label.

NOTES:

6

VISITING THE SALON

There are basically two kinds of hairdressers: ones who care about how your hair *looks* (stylists) and ones who care about your *hair* (healthy hairdressers). Hopefully, you already have a wonderful healthy hairdresser to work with. Talented, reliable hairdressers are not easy to find, so when you find someone who will work with you, stay with them. It's best to work with someone who knows your hair and listens to your input. Whoever you work with should respect your decision to focus on the health of your hair and make changes accordingly. But what do you do if you don't have a reliable hairdresser?

Finding a good salon is not easy. I have moved around a lot, and have had some bad experiences while trying to find a new Healthy Hair Partner. Or, I would find a talented hairdresser, only to have my time disrespected. You may have had some of the same experiences. However, your Healthy Hair Partner *is* out there.

YOUR HEALTHY HAIR PARTNER

Whether it's a relaxer, a deep conditioner or bothersom scalp problem, taking care of your hair sometimes requires professional help. That help should be your Healthy Hair Partner. A Healthy Hair Partner can be a hairdresser, stylist or friend who has a 'knack' with hair — basically someone who can put in a proper perm for you, help you recognize potential problems, recommend solutions and offer advice.

If your Partner is at a salon, be sure to take your hair diary when visiting them. Most of us only see our hairdresser every month or so, so taking your diary with you can help them identify potential problems. In your diary, list what products, medications or perms you used. Most hairdressers will keep a file on your hair; you should keep one as well. Use your diary to write down questions, hairstyle ideas, suggestions or anything else you might want to discuss with your Partner. Doing so will make sure you do not forget once you get in the chair. You can also use your diary to list your hairdresser's phone number, email and address if they change salons or move.

Don't be afraid to talk openly with your Partner. Often, when hairdressers say, "Do you like your hair?" we say yes, then comb out our hair the minute we leave. And on top of that, give them a tip! Hairdressers are professionals, and want to provide you with a service and style you are happy with. So speak up!

There are some things to keep in mind when choosing a new Hair Partner or salon. Time is one — will you have to wait an hour before you are seen or spend five hours in the salon? A properly scheduled perm, trim and roller set should only take two or three hours. The salon itself should be clean, including the sink, chair, and floor and styling tools. Don't ever be afraid to speak up or make suggestions! Fortunately, there are many professional salons that provide excellent customer service.

Here are some ways to find a good hairdresser in your area:

1. **Network.** Talk to everyone, and I do mean every one! If you see a lady at the mall with beautiful hair, ask who does her hair. Focus on people whose hair is shiny and healthy looking. Most people are eager to help and will either rave about their favorite salon, or vehemently rant about the ones to avoid. Always ask for the stylist's first and last name to make sure you go to the right person. Inquire about what products they use at the salon, and the average price for a relaxer.

2. **Surf.** Visit hairoil.com, blackpages.com, everythingblack. com, blackvoices.com, longhaircareforum.com, blackhairmedia.com or city search guides to find good salons in your area.

3. **Discount hair salons.** Don't turn your nose up at BoRics,® Hair Cuttery® or SuperCuts.® Most of these salons have some Black stylists and an informal atmosphere. Talk to them to get a feel for their skill level and hair philosophy. Discount hair salons usually give you a choice of products that may include Nexxus® and Affirm.® They also incorporate an a la carte system of choosing services, which is great if you are limited in time or money.

4. **Department stores.** JCPenney,® Marshall Fields® and even Wal-Mart® have excellent salons. These salons employ outstanding, talented stylists in a convenient location. Also, they may stay open later and are open on weekends, including Sundays.

CHEMICAL RELAXERS

There are two different ways to get a relaxer: virgin and touch-up.

Virgin relaxers are procedures in which the entire head of hair is chemically straightened. Most of us will only get one virgin perm in our lifetime. Once the hair has been chemically straightened, it does not revert or need to be straightened again. During a touch-up, the relaxer is only applied to the new growth (hair that has not yet been relaxed). Properly applied relaxers will not over-lap, allowing the hair to retain its elasticity and strength.

A **perm cycle** is the length of time between perms. Each perm cycle should be at least 7–8 weeks long to allow adequate hair growth and discourage over-processing. However, do not wait longer than ten weeks to get your hair relaxed. Doing so may put extra tension on the hair where the new hair and processed hair meet and may even result in breakage.

Tip: Never let anyone spread the relaxer creme all the way to the ends. This almost guarantees breakage.

GETTING THE KINKS OUT

There are three kinds of chemical relaxers: no-base with **sodium hydroxide** (lye), based with **guanidine hydroxide** (no-lye) and ammonium thioglycolate. At the time of this writing, there are no effective "natural" hair relaxers.

Lye or sodium hydroxide relaxers are the strongest kind of perm. Lye perms have a pH level of 12–14. Sodium hydroxide is a caustic type of chemical that penetrates into the cortex (inner layer) of the hair shaft and breaks the cross-bonds, causing the hair to relax, or straighten. I have been using lye perms more than ten years with great success.

Guanidine hydroxide relaxers are a mix of calcium hydroxide and guanidine carbonate and have a lower pH than lye perms, between 10–12. Guanidine hydroxide relaxers are referred to as no-lye relaxers. Many sensitive scalp relaxers are no-lye perms because they are thought to be less damaging than sodium hydroxide relaxers but these perms can still damage the hair and scalp. During the relaxer process, calcium in the relaxer is deposited onto the hair. This build-up over time can make your dry, brittle or frizzy. Some women complain that their hair feels more coarse and dry after a no lye perm and attribute the resulting breakage to their use.

Tip: Once you start with a no-lye perm, you must stick with it, or grow your hair out then cut off the previously relaxed hair.

Choosing a relaxer type is a personal choice; some do well with one kind while others do well with another. When getting a relaxer, make sure you understand what type of perm is being used, then make a note of how your hair feels afterward. It should be straight and shiny, not dry or hard. If it is, or if you are experiencing breakage even after using the hair regimen in this book, you are probably using the wrong kind of perm for your hair.

Many Caucasian women and men use **ammonium thioglyco-late**-based relaxers to remove the curl from their hair. Ammonium thioglycolate perms are advertised as being less permanent than sodium hydroxide and guanidine hydroxide-based perms. Because they work a little differently than the others (they relax hair by making changes to the cystine [protein] linkage) ammonium thio-glycolate perms do not work well on Black hair. With a pH of 9.0–9.5, these are also considered to be less damaging, yet still require a neutralization step to restore the hair's natural pH level.

Keep in mind that all relaxer cremes are not created equal. Each manufacturer has its own formula; relaxer may have the same *ingredients* but not in the same *quantities* (some are stronger than others). When you find a brand that work for you, stick with it.

Making the Appointment

When you make an appointment to receive a relaxer, make sure you specify whether you will need a virgin, or a touch-up. Inquire about the kinds of products used and what they cost. Most salons will charge extra for deep conditioners, hair trims, and semi-permanent hair colors. Ask to speak to the stylist directly and if your hair is damaged request a **consultation**. During the consultation, which may or may not occur at the same time as your service, the stylist will check the condition of your hair and scalp. S/he will check for dandruff, evaluate the elasticity of your hair and should ask you to fill out a history form or client profile. Use this time to ask any questions you may have. Write them down prior to your appointment and take them with you.

Before the Appointment

Prior to your appointment (72–48 hours), wash your hair with a clarifying or build-up removing shampoo to allow the perm better penetration. Do not use gel, undiluted setting lotion or hair spray when styling as your scalp and hair should be clean. Do not fall into the "you get a better perm with dirty hair" myth. If your hair has a layer of dirt and build-up on it, the relaxer has to pene-trate through that first, which will make the straightening process take longer. Also, a dirty scalp will itch, tempting you to scratch.

During the 24 hours prior to your appointment, keep scalp and hair manipulation to a bare minimum. Eliminating excess hair combing, scalp massages and brushing will keep your scalp intact. Many times, because we know we can't scratch, our scalp will begin to itch. Resist the temptation, but if really have an itch, pat your head or gently rub where it itches (on top of your hair) in a circular motion. If for any reason you suffer a scrape or cut on your scalp prior to your service, reschedule your appointment.

The day of your appointment, arrive on time or a few minutes early to guarantee your spot in the chair. If you scratch or burn easily, ask to have your scalp protected or based. Make sure the hairdresser uses a petroleum-based product or solution designed specifically for this use. Your ears and hairline should be pro-tected as well.

Should You Perm Your Hair Yourself?

I do not recommend relaxing your own hair for several reasons. You cannot see the back of your head to apply the perm properly, there is a higher possibility of over-lapping and there is a higher risk to you. Chemical strighteners contain dangerous chemicals that can cause blindness or death if ingested. I know some of you may feel confident enough to perm your hair yourself, but leave this process to the professionals.

If you do decide to perm your hair yourself, be sure to take the following precautions:

1. **Make sure you have time set aside** with no interruptions. Turn off the phone and ensure the kids are asleep or taken care of.

2. **Always use gloves** to protect your hands and wear clear plastic safety glasses to protect your eyes.

3. **Protect your scalp and hairline** with petroleum or relaxer base.

4. **Use an egg timer** for processing time.

5. **Use care not to over-lap** or over-process your hair. Try protecting your processed hair with a light layer of base or conditioner.

6. **Apply the relaxer with an applicator brush or the back of a fine tooth comb.** These tools will give you better control of the relaxer creme and help you smooth it in.

7. **Use a quality product.** Try Affirm® by Avalon, Designer Touch,® Vitale® and Mizani® relaxers.

8. **Shampoo at least three times with a neutralizing shampoo** and rinse thoroughly. You may need to ask someone to help to ensure all of the perm is removed.

HAIR TRIMS

Our hair grows at an average rate of ½ inch a month. A good trim should not take off more than ¼ inch, just enough to maintain your shape and cut off split ends. A split end (**fragilitas crinium**) is what occurs when a hair breaks or is damaged. Once the hair shaft is split, it must be trimmed off. Conditioners can "glue" your hair back together temporarily but if the end is not trimmed, it will continue to split and eventually break. I have seen some hair strands on my own head that have split three and four times! Hair that is not treated well should be trimmed every other relaxer or three times a year. However, if you treat your hair well, there is no need to sacrifice your length by getting your hair trimmed after every perm. Contrary to popular belief, cutting your hair will not make it grow. If you avoid direct heat and handle your hair with care, trim your hair as infrequently as every six months, or every second or third perm.

Should You Trim Your Hair Yourself?

There is nothing more frustrating that asking for a trim and getting butchered. I cried the last time someone cut layers in my hair and I specifically asked for a trim (don't tell anybody). However, there is nothing like a good, professional haircut. Talk to your stylist and be specific about how much will be cut. Watch them in a mirror if necessary.

You can cut your own hair, or ask a friend you trust to do it for you. If you want to trim your hair yourself, purchase a pair of professional hair cutting scissors from a beauty supply store. They are expensive, but you can find a pair for less than ten dollars. It is best to trim your hair while it is dry and straight (after a fresh perm). To trim your hair, simply comb your hair straight up or down and lightly snip off the ends. Don't worry about getting your hair even; leave that for the professionals. You just want to clean off any split or damaged ends.

What if Your Hair is Damaged?

Because truly damaged hair has no way to repair itself, you have to decide whether you want to start anew or if you want to try to work with what you have. I used to beg my girlfriend Jacqueline to let me trim her hair. She had a mushroom hair cut that was about two inches longer in one spot, but nothing I said or did would make her cut it. One day she finally acquiesced, and was surprised and pleased at the results. Her attitude and fear of losing her hair had to be addressed, but what she didn't realize was that she was killing her hair by allowing the ends to continually break. Sometimes, when you try to hard to hold onto something, you end up losing it anyway.

If your hair is in bad shape, ask yourself the following questions:

1. Has your breakage stopped or slowed down?

2. Does a professional wash and deep conditioning leave your hair looking and feeling good?

3. Is your hair uneven due to excessive breakage?

4. Is it damaged due to mistreatment or over-processing?

If you answered yes to questions 1 and 2 it should be possible to salvage what you have. Get a trim and move forward. However, every situation is different. If you answered yes to both 3 and 4, your situation is more severe and you will need a good haircut to even your hair out. Don't worry; your hair will grow back! The following chapters will show you how.

NOTES:

_____

_____

_____

_____

7

MAINTAINING YOUR HAIR

To maintain your hair, we will take everything we've learned and expand on it. You should have all your supplies, a good understanding of the hair growth process and know how to care for a healthy scalp. Now let's put it all into action.

HEALTHY HAIR REGIMEN

- Wash hair and deep condition (with or without heat) hair twice a week

- Use a protein treatment once a perm cycle

- No heat styling

- Protect your hair

- Regular relaxers every 7–9 weeks

- Hair trims 2–3 times per year

- Semi-permanent hair color only

- Oil ends and hairline every night

- Take a Break once or twice a year

WASH AND DEEP CONDITION

Commit to washing your hair twice a week. Why so often? Believe it or not, your hair grows faster when it's clean. Dirt, oil, product build-up and pollutants can dry your hair and make your scalp itch. A good shampoo will clean and invigorate your scalp and help restore your hair to its normal pH level (4.5–5.5). Wash your hair every four days or sooner if it starts to feel dry.

Another reason for frequent washing is that relaxed hair needs extra moisture. 90% of this moisture will come from your deep conditioner, especially when applied with heat. The remainder will come from your leave-in conditioner and hair oil. Did you ever notice how your hair is longer when it's wet? That is because it has absorbed so much water that hair shaft becomes swollen and has begun to stretch. Wouldn't it make sense that some of that water would be retained after the hair is dry? Contrary to popular belief, washing does not dry your hair out, heat and chemicals do!

When heat is used on our hair, it dries out even more quickly; blow-drying alone can take most of the moisture out of our hair. Hair that is washed infrequently quickly becomes dehydrated and brittle.

But what if you oil your hair every day? Do you still need to wash twice a week? The answer is yes! We know that our hair is porous, like a sponge. Have you ever tried to wipe up oil with an old, dry sponge? It doesn't work well; the oil we add to our hair needs water to be absorbed! Also, oil is thicker than water and takes up more room in the hair shaft. Our hair can only absorb so much and the rest will simply build-up on the hair shaft, make your hair look greasy and create dandruff.

I recommend that you choose specific days and keep a regular schedule. For instance, you could wash your hair on Saturday night and then again on Wednesday night. Think of these nights as your beauty nights, when you take care of you.

SAMPLE HAIR WEEK

• Sunday: Wash and deep condition hair

• Monday: Oil hairline and ends, style hair without heat

• Tuesday: Oil hairline and ends, wear hair up to protect the ends

• Wednesday: Wash and deep condition hair

• Thursday: Oil hairline and ends, style hair without heat

• Friday: Oil hairline and ends, style hair without heat

• Saturday: Oil hairline and ends, wear hair up to protect the ends

• Sunday: Wash and deep condition hair

How to Wash Your Hair

Make sure you have the following supplies handy:

• Shampoo for your hair type

• Deep conditioner

• Light conditioner

• Wide tooth comb

• Fine tooth comb

• Hair oil

• Leave-in conditioner

• Shine or gloss

• Plastic cap

When washing your hair, it is best if you get in the shower. You may give yourself a back-ache and won't be able to rinse properly if you wash your hair in the sink. Start by rinsing your hair to remove any leave-in conditioner or styling aids. Use a quarter-sized dollop of shampoo and rub your hands together to distribute it. Put the shampoo on your scalp, not the ends of your hair. Work up a lather by massaging your scalp with your fingers and scalp brush. Don't mix your hair all over your head; the more you do, the more tangled it will become.

You may notice that during the first shampoo, you won't have much lather. That is because your hair is still dirty! Rinse well and then repeat, but this time, let the shampoo sit for a minute (especially if you are using a protein shampoo). Rinse, then press the water out of your hair. Never squeeze or pull your hair when it's wet. Instead, smooth your hands down from the top of your head down to remove excess water. If your hair is longer, gather your hair at the base of your neck with one hand, and once anchored, use the other hand to gently press the water out of the ends of your hair.

Hot or Cold Water?

Honestly, it doesn't matter because the effects are barely noticeable. However, experts say to wash hair in hot or warm water to help remove dirt and build-up and to rinse hair in cool water to close the cuticle and add shine.

Deep Conditioning

Conditioners penetrate better on towel dried hair so remove excess water first. Then, use a generous amount (half-dollar size dollop or more for longer hair) to make sure the hair is completely covered. Concentrate on your hairline, nape and the ends of your hair, where it's needed most. Massage well, but DO NOT COMB THROUGH. Snap on a plastic cap and sit under a warm dryer for 10 minutes. Rinse well and follow with an instant conditioner.

Tip: Add a teaspoon of Shea butter or a few drops of your hair oil to your conditioner for extra conditioning.

PROTEIN TREATMENTS

As we discussed in Chapter 5, a liquid protein treatment can strengthen your hair and arrest breakage almost immediately. The protein is infused onto the hair using heat and the results should last for about six weeks. Use this treatment the week after your relaxer to help repair some of the damage from the chemicals (the chemicals will remove the protein layer as well). Protein treatments are powerful; their use must be taken very seriously. Be sure you read the instructions completely before using. If you do not feel comfortable doing a lot to your hair, you can have this procedure done at the salon.

How to Apply a Protein Treatment

If you are using Aphoghees® Protein Treatment, apply the treatment after shampooing or according to the instructions. To ease application, divide your hair into four sections first. Then, pour a small amount of the product into your hand and apply the conditioner to each section of your hair. Concentrate on your ends and hairline; do not manipulate your hair unnecessarily or comb the conditioner through. When your entire head is covered, pile your hair on top of your head (do not use clips) and process under a warm dryer for 10 minutes without a plastic cap. Rinse well and follow with the accompanying moisturizing treatment.

As your hair becomes healthier, you may notice that it is starting to feel hard or coarse. This is good news; it means your hair is getting stronger. If this happens, simply cut down on the protein treatments to once every other perm cycle or try a lighter version like Nexxus Emergencee.® To use Emergencee,® apply it after your shampoo. Cover with a plastic cap and process under the dryer for 10 minutes.

SAMPLE PERM CYCLE

• Week 1: Perm, no trim

• Week 2: Wash and use protein treatment

• Week 2: Wash and deep condition

• Week 3: Wash and deep condition twice

• Week 4: Wash and deep condition twice

• Week 5: Wash and deep condition twice

• Week 6: Wash and deep condition twice

• Week 7: Wash and deep condition

• Week 7: Wash with a clarifying shampoo and condition, style without gel

• Week 8: Perm, with trim

• Week 9: Wash and use protein treatment

NO HEAT STYLING

Blow dryers, flat irons and curling irons change your hair's shape by using high temperatures to soften your hair's keratin structure. Styling your hair with heat reduces its moisture level and leaves it weak and susceptible to damage. Using heat on damaged hair is twice as bad; heat can penetrate through broken cuticles scales to access the cortex even faster.

I have not used a blow dryer for more than ten years and cannot remember the last time I used a curling iron. It is possible to regularly style your hair without heat. Chapter 12 will show you how.

Some women fall into the trap of over-using curling irons because of convenience. You can prevent unnecessary damage to your hair by planning ahead. Wrap your hair well or add a few curlers at night to avoid using a curling iron during the morning rush.

To use heat wisely, remember these rules:

• Save its use for emergencies and special occasions.

• Always test the level of heat prior to using the appliance. Keep a damp rag near by to test the temperature. If it sizzles, it's too hot!

• Water conducts heat, so never use hair sprays or curl wet hair.

• Always add a few drops of oil to your hair before blow-drying and again before curling. The oil provides a protective layer and will burn off.

• Always use a medium setting.

• Never hold the curling iron in place for more than three seconds.

• Dry your hair and scalp under a hooded dryer or let it dry naturally before blow-drying.

• Keep the blow dryer moving constantly. Don't concentrate heat in one spot.

• Whenever possible, avoid the added damage of blow-drying your hair and then using a hot iron. Use curling irons or flat irons on hair that has been wrapped or roller set.

SALON SERVICES

Whether you go to the salon or apply your relaxers at home, be sure to get them regularly. Dermatologists have stated that six weeks in between perms is too frequent.[2] Therefore, the minimum amount of time between perms should be at least 7–8 weeks to allow adequate hair growth.

Avoid permanent colors at all costs! Permanent colors process your hair using hydrogen peroxide and ammonia. Our hair is *already* processed and double-processing your hair will almost guarantee breakage. If you want to cover gray hair, use a semi-permanent hair color, or **rinse.** Hair rinses are temporary and can be applied the same day as a relaxer. If you have them applied on the same day, the color will penetrate deeper and the results will be darker and last longer. Choose a semi-permanent color that is **Level 1, deposit only.** Be careful; some colors say they are semi-permanent but contain peroxide. If you have to mix anything, it's not for you.

Recommendations:

- Jazzing®

- Beautiful Browns by Clairol®

- Sebastian Colourshines by Cellophanes.®

If you simply must lighten your hair, consider getting a few highlights. Highlights are damaging as well, but because they are only applied in specific areas the damage is not as significant. You should have your highlights applied by a professional color expert, however, if you want to try this at home, use a plastic highlight cap with a semi-permanent hair color, like Nice 'n Easy.® Do not use bleach or highlighting kits. Try applying a rinse over highlights for a dramatic effect.

PROTECTING YOUR INVESTMENT

One of the most important parts of any healthy hair regimen is protecting your hair from damage. Even the healthiest of hair must be protected to remain healthy. First and foremost, protect those ends! As your hair grows, retaining the ends is what makes your hair become longer. Protect your ends by keeping them moisturized and wearing a protective hairstyle. Adding a few drops of oil to your hair ends each day will help keep your hair supple and flexible. Wear your hair up in a French roll or bun as often as possible and get into the habit of wearing your hair up in a protective hairstyle after a few days of wearing it down. If you club or go out a lot, wear you hair up during the week for school or work, and wear your hair down on the weekend. I rarely wear my hair down; it's either in a sleek ponytail or French roll.

Sample Hair Day

• Morning: Oil hairline and ends, style hair without heat

• Night: Oil hairline and ends, tie hair up

Some other ways your hair can be damaged include:

Harsh Styling

Using a wide tooth comb and handling your hair with care will protect its cuticle layer. Natural bristle or boar bristle brushes are NOT to be used because the tightly packed bristles are much too rough on relaxed hair; use your cushioned paddle brush (wide bristles) instead.

Wet or dry, your hair must be treated with care. Never tug through tangles or brush hair while wet. When styling, always use a wide tooth comb. If you need to do detailed styling, use your wide tooth comb *first*, then follow with a fine tooth comb. And remember, avoid backcombing or "ratting" your hair.

Heat

You can protect your hair from heat by simply avoiding it or limiting its use. Heat can burn your hair and rob it of precious moisture. Never use a curling iron or pressing comb at a temperature higher than 150°. Never curl wet hair or use hair spray with a curling iron. For more information refer to the section "using heat wisely" on page 61.

UV Rays

Harmful Ultraviolet (UV) rays can damage your skin and hair. UV rays affect the cuticle in a way similar to bleach by penetrating the cuticle layer; prolonged exposure will lighten and dry your hair. You can protect your hair by covering it with sunscreen (the kind for your skin) or using a leave-in conditioner with sunscreen. Also, wear a hat when in direct sunlight.

Wool Coats, Sweaters, Cotton Pillowcases and Scarves

Friction from wool coats, sweater and turtlenecks can cause breakage. You can protect your hair by wearing nylon coats, wearing your hair up while wearing turtlenecks or covering wool coats with a silk scarf. The best way to protect your hair at night is to tie it up. If you toss and turn a lot while sleeping wear a satin bonnet and tie a long scarf around the hairline to help hold it in place. Using a satin pillow case can help during those times when your scarf refuses to stay put.

Cosmetics and Facial Cleansers

Because the hair around your hairline is thin it needs extra protection. The hair follicles in that area are less dense (fewer per inch) than in other areas so hair loss in this area will quickly become noticeable. You can protect your hairline with a barrier of heavy hair oil or grease. Use it morning and night to prevent facial wash, face lotions and cosmetics from getting in your hair and drying it out.

NOTES:

8

GIVE YOUR HAIR A BREAK!

Our hair can become stressed for a multitude of reasons, just as we can. A Break is a vacation for your hair and it's extreme: absolutely no heat, chemicals (other than a relaxer) or every day combing and styling. A Break also involves wearing your hair in a protective hairstyle for an extended period of time. Your Break hairstyle should hold your hair in place, protect your ends and remove the need to comb and style it on a daily basis. Good examples are braids, cornrows and ponytails. During your Break, as your hair grows, the ends are retained and you hair becomes longer. Therefore, the longer the Break, the longer your hair will be. I recommend that women who want long hair give their hair a Break for a full 12 weeks (or two perm cycles) to revive their hair and accelerate growth. Then, to maintain healthy hair, take a Break at least once a year for an entire perm cycle (time in between perms). What you are doing isn't revolutionary; it's what you *aren't* doing that makes it work.

Take your Break *very* seriously; don't overlook its importance. They take time and can get boring (believe me, I know) but stick it out. I believe this was the single most important thing I did for my hair; they will make a significant difference in the length and condition of your hair. During your Break, instead of focusing on your hair style, use this time to start a new exercise program (it won't matter if you sweat your hair out) or other personal goal. After your six weeks are up you can show off your new body and your new 'do!

I usually get medium size individual braids and will wear them for up to eight weeks. By the end of my Break I am so excited to wear my hair down and am always amazed at how much longer and healthier my hair is.

BRAIDS

Braids are fantastic ways to escalate your hair growth. They work in a couple of different ways: 1. the hair is physically protected; 2. no heat and no daily styling prevents damage to your hair; 3. braid mists keep your hair's moisture level balanced; and 4. the pressure from properly input braids can help keep your scalp stimulated.

Shorter hair is maintained best in braids. However, braids work wonders regardless of hair length. Have your braids put in at least two weeks after your perm to allow some new growth to come in. The day of or night before getting braids, prepare your hair and scalp by washing and deep conditioning your hair, then use a leave-in conditioner. Applying Scalpacin® or other prescription anti–itch medicine on your scalp can work wonders to prevent itching.

Getting Braids

Use a recommended braider or someone whose work you have seen. Many people do them out of their homes and can offer a reduced price, but make certain the braider understands that you will continue to wear a relaxer. Some African salons don't understand the tension braids put on relaxed hair and do things that are unhealthy to relaxed hair. For instance, never let your braider sweep a flame across the braid to "seal" it (only the ends should be sealed; see next section).

Your braids should be tight enough to be secure, but not overly so. This light pressure should be similar to hair tugging (see page 87) and may help keep your scalp stimulated for a while. However, too much pressure may harm your hair; there should not be more than ¼ inch of scalp showing between braids. The braids should not stress your scalp; this is a time of rest for your hair and scalp.

What Kind of Braids Should I Get?

Large braids or cornrows are the preferred style. They offer the most protection, are easiest to care for and last the longest, but stay away from micro-braids. Cornrows should be re-done on a weekly or bi-weekly basis but individual braids can be worn for up to eight weeks. Shorter hair can have the ends sealed (burned) but longer hair should use rubber bands to avoid cutting your own hair during removal.

Maintaining Your Braids

To keep your braids moisturized and smelling good, use a homemade braid mist.

Braid Mist

- ¾ cup water

- ¼ cup natural oil (almond, olive, etc)

- 20–25 drops of your favorite essential oil

   Store in a spray bottle; shake well before using.

   Remember, your hair will dry out after a few days and the mois-ture needs to be replenished. The oil and water in your braid mist will be absorbed by your hair and scalp and will help keep it sup-ple. Avoid using store bought braid sprays because they can leave a build-up on your braids which is extremely difficult to remove. Tea tree oil can be used on your scalp if necessary to relieve itch-ing. Don't worry about washing your braids; your braid mist will supply moisture to your hair, and it is too difficult to rinse all of the shampoo out of your braids. If you go swimming, just rinse your hair well, then apply instant conditioner. Let it sit for a few minutes and rinse again. Remove excess water by pressing them with a towel; but don't rub them or they will begin to look frizzy.

> Tip: Do not put anything on your braids except your braid mist or conditioner.

Removing Your Braids

   To remove individual braids, enlist some help. This process can take 2–3 times as long as it took to put them in. When removing braid hair, undo the braid; never pull the hair out. There may be a clump of dandruff, hair and build-up at the bottom of your hair near your scalp. To remove it, just spray some Ultra Sheen® or Stay Soft Fro® on it, and then rub it in. Use a medium tooth comb to gently loosen and remove the build-up. Repeat this process on each braid. Then, wash your hair using a super detangling shampoo such as Cream of Nature,® deep condition and style as usual.

Cornrows can simply be unbraided and washed. Because they are redone so frequently, there should not be any build-up.

SLICKED TO THE SIDE

If you choose not to wear braids, your Break style should lay flat on your head and sides so it is easy to wrap up at night and maintain. Keep in mind that during your Break, you will *not* be styling your hair. If you think will be tempted after a few weeks to style or wear your hair down, get braids instead.

I watched my girlfriend Grace grow her hair without missing a beat. Grace had a short, close-cropped hairstyle that looked great but, when she got married, her husband challenged her to grow her hair. She did, and always wore the cutest styles. When Grace's hair was about to her ears she would part it on one side and slick her hair low across her forehead behind her other ear. The other side was slicked down behind her ear. Her hair in the back was laid flat.

How to Get This Style

This one is a snap. Wash your hair first, then condition and detangle with your wide tooth comb. Next, use your fine tooth comb to part your hair and comb into your desired shape. Apply the desired amount of protein gel with your fingers to cover and protect your hair; however, don't put so much in that it will begin to flake and crack. Use the back of your comb to smooth out wrinkles and create waves. Dry naturally or under the dryer. It's as easy as that!

Another option is do finger waves. Not old school finger waves, just a slight wave pattern to make your hair look pretty. There's no need to sacrifice your style; add headbands and barrettes to jazz up your look. Experiment with makeup to make your eyes stand out or get a sexy new lipstick color to go along with this elegant style.

Maintaining This Style

Your daily grooming routine should now be short and sweet. Just untie your wrap, and smooth your edges, but don't comb your hair down or re-part your hair. Reapply protein gel as needed or a little water to reactivate the gel. At night, be sure to add some hair oil to your hairline and tie it back up again; a must or this style will break and get messy.

PONYTAILS

A lot of hairdressers frown on the frequent use of a ponytail fearing damage to their clients' hair. However, this style is versatile and can be protective if done properly. The trick is to make sure your ponytail is not pulled too tightly and to protect your ends.

Getting a Ponytail

After washing, conditioning and detangling your hair (be sure to use leave-in conditioner), comb it into a ponytail and gather your hair either at the base of your neck or at the top of your head (for drawstring ponytails). Use your fine tooth comb to gently remove any remaining tangles and part your hair. Once your hair is in the style you want. use protein gel to smooth it out and hold it down. You can apply the gel with your fingers or with a fine tooth comb, then fasten your hair with a ponytail holder. The ponytail should be secure but don't damage your hair by pulling it too tight. Cover the ends of your hair with gel as well. If you are wearing a braid or phony-pony add it at this time. Dry your hair under the dryer or let it air-dry.

Removing the Ponytail

If you are wearing a piece, remove it gently, then remove the ponytail holder by untying it completely; never pull it off your hair. Rinse your hair well to remove styling aids then wash and condition. When detangling your hair don't be alarmed at the amount of hair loss. Remember, you lose 75–100 hairs a day. Depending on how long you had your hair up you will see all of the hair that was shed during that time. If is has been four days expect to see 300-400 hairs, on average. Finish detangling with your fine tooth comb and repeat the process above.

SUMMARY

Challenge yourself! See how long you can stay on your Break. Set a coming out date on which you will show off your longer, healthier locks.

Whatever your style, remember; it should not involve any heat and should protect the ends of your hair. Your Break hairstyle should not require any daily combing or fluffing to look good. It is for this reason that I don't recommend French rolls during a Break but, a French roll is an excellent healthy hairstyle. To achieve a good looking French roll you will need to do styling that should be avoided during your Break. Keep it simple!

NOTES:

_____

_____

_____

_____

_____

_____

_____

_____

_____

_____

_____

_____

_____

9

VITAMINS, MINERALS AND NUTRITIONAL SUPPLEMENTS

Now that we know how to take care of our hair from the outside, let's learn how to take care of it from the inside. Hair loss, dry hair and an itchy scalp can be caused by a vitamin deficiency, crash diet and even stress. You need a nutritious, balanced diet to grow healthy hair. Crash diets and junk foods rob your hair of precious nutrients. Eating a sensible diet of carbohydrates, protein and good fats combined with a daily multivitamin will help you and your hair glow. But before we go any further, let's get one thing straight: there is no magic pill to make your hair grow. However, there are some nutrients that are essential to healthy hair growth:

Supplement	Type	RDA	You Need
Biotin	B vitamin	300 mcg	600–1200 mcg
Folic Acid	B vitamin	400 mg	400–800 mg
Iron	mineral	15 mg	15–27 mg
Vitamin C	antioxidant	60mg	500–1500 mg
Zinc	mineral	12 mg	20–30 mg
Protein	amino acid	.8 mg/kg body weight	1 mg/kg body weight
Essential Fatty Acids	fatty acid	N/A	1000–3000mg

RDA = Recommended Daily Allowance;
Mcg – microgram 1000 = 1 mg
Mg – milligram 1000 = 1 gram

All of these nutrients complement each other. For instance, Vitamin C helps the body absorb iron and protein while essential fatty acids help the body absorb zinc.

Tip: Talk to your doctor before adding any supplements to your diet or embarking on any weight reduction program.

Biotin is a water-soluble (dissolves in water) B vitamin used in the production of proteins that is required for healthy hair, skin and nails. Biotin is sometimes called Vitamin H. Foods that are rich in biotin include beef liver, egg yolk, nuts, whole grains and brewers yeast.

RDA: 300 mcg
You need: 600–1200 mcg

Folate (folic acid) is another form of the B vitamin that is needed for cell replication and hair growth. Folic acid helps feed active cells that wear out and divide quickly, like hair and skin cells. Leafy green vegetables such as spinach and turnip greens, dry beans and peas, fortified cereals and grain products are rich in folic acid. Pregnant women and those who take birth control pills need extra folic acid.

RDA: 400 mcg daily

You need: 400 mcg–800 mcg

NOTE: A variety of prescription drugs including antacids, anti-cancer drugs, and anticonvulsants interfere with the absorption of folic acid.

Iron, an essential mineral, is an important component of proteins. Iron is also required to produce hemoglobin, the oxygen-carrying component of the blood. Hemoglobin helps your hair grow by bringing oxygen to your hair follicles. Women with heavy monthly periods can lose a significant amount of iron and may be deficient. Iron can be found in meats, fish, beans, and enriched flour, cereal, and grain products.

RDA: 15 mg

You need: 15–27 mg

Tip: If you think you are iron deficient see your doctor for medical diagnosis and treatment. Don't take more then 27 mg of iron without a prescription. Take iron with vitamin C (orange juice) to aid with absorption. Iron may cause constipation.

Vitamin C, or ascorbic acid, is an antioxidant that helps your body destroy free radicals (atoms with an odd number of electrons that cause aging and some cancers). Vitamin C is essential for healthy blood vessels, muscles, gums, bones and teeth, and is involved in the production of collagen, a protein necessary for healthy skin and hair.

RDA: 60 mg

You need: 500–1500 mg

Tip:
Smokers need extra Vitamin C.

Zinc is an essential mineral found in almost every cell, including hair. It synthesizes protein, helps cells reproduce, and stimulates the activity of enzymes (substances that promote biochemical reactions in your body). Children with alopecia areata (patchy areas of hair loss) have been reported to be deficient in zinc. Foods that are rich in zinc include oysters, meat, eggs, seafood, fortified breakfast cereals, black-eyed peas, tofu, nuts and whole grains.

RDA: 12 mg

You need: 20 mg–30mg

PROTEIN

We learned earlier that hair is composed of dead protein cells. Protein is used in the body to build tissues, as an energy source and to grow, repair and maintain your hair. Lean meats including turkey and chicken, eggs and fish are excellent sources of protein. If you are a vegetarian, you may not be getting enough protein. You can increase your intake of protein by eating more nuts, tofu and beans. Also, consider adding a protein shake to your diet.

Amino acids are the building blocks of protein. **Arginine** and **cysteine** are amino acids used by the hair follicles to build hair. Amino acids can be supplied in supplement form or from your protein source.

RDA: 0.8mg per kg of weight

You need: 1mg per kg of weight

To calculate: divide your weight by 2.2. The result is your weight in kilograms (kg) and is how much protein you need.

Example:

Weight 150 lbs

150/2.2=68

68 grams of protein daily

MULTI-VITAMINS

Most people could benefit from taking a daily multi-vitamin. Why? Because we don't eat as well as we think we do. Even if you do eat 4–6 servings of fruits and vegetables each day, preparing them may destroy much of their nutritional content. Microwaves kill vitamins and minerals, as do hot water and high heat. Therefore, there is no way to accurately determine if we are actually getting the Recommended Daily Allowance (RDA) of nutritional elements required.

We need the RDA just to exist, but we need more than that to grow healthy hair. Most of the vitamins your hair needs are water soluble, meaning the body cannot store them and the excess will be excreted. These vitamins must be replenished daily. Taking supplements of biotin, for example, will help rid your body of an existing deficiency as well as meeting its daily need. Vitamin deficiencies are not created overnight, so we can't expect them to be resolved immediately. It may be necessary to take a supplement for 4–6 months to overcome a deficiency. One of the benefits of hair vitamins is they include a good mix of nutrients which can significantly cut down on the number of pills you take each day. I find that the more pills we take, the less we want to take them! It is possible, however, to get the nutrients your hair needs from a regular multi-vitamin and supplement the rest. Therefore, when choosing a multi-vitamin, read the labels! Look for one that supplies most of the 50 essential vitamins and minerals.

Tip: When reading vitamin labels, check the serving size to find out how many pills the amounts are based on. For instance, many supplements require you take 2 or even 3 pills to provide the amount listed on the bottle.

Recommendations:

- GNC,® Women's Ultra Nourish Hair

- GNC,® Women's Hair, Skin & Nails Formula

- GNC,® Nourish Hair

- One Source,® Women's daily

Tip: Take your supplements with meals. If you take more than one, take one with each meal.

ESSENTIAL FATTY ACIDS

In addition to your daily multi-vitamin, I recommend that you supplement your diet with the essential fatty acids (EFA) alpha lineolenic acid (ALA) and gamma linoliec acid (GLA). Also known as the healthy fats, EFAs are an important part of your healthy hair diet. EFAs play a crucial role in the health and beauty of your hair and scalp by providing them with lubrication from the inside. They are essential, meaning they cannot be made in the body and must be eaten or supplemented to avoid deficiencies. Studies have shown that, ALA can relieve dandruff and GLA can benefit eczema, stop hair loss and moisturize dry hair.[3] Your body needs both but, depending on your particular hair problems, you can supplement with one or the other.

Gamma Linoliec Acid (GLA) is part of the Omega 6 fatty acid family. Evening primrose oil is an excellent source of GLA (45mg per 500 mg capsule). I take 3000 milligrams of evening primrose oil daily. Studies have shown that evening primrose oil can relieve a host of ailments, including PMS, high blood pressure, obesity and high cholesterol.[4] This supplement is especially important if you suffer from hair loss or take thyroid medication.

Alpha lineolenic acid is an Omega 3 fatty acid. Studies have shown that ALA is especially beneficial for skin and scalp problems including dandruff and eczema and may even lower bad cholesterol.[5] Flax seed oil is an excellent source of ALA, containing about 540mg of ALA per gram. Flax seed oil is unique in that it contains a small amount of GLA as well, about 129 mg per gram.

Tip: Store your EFA in the refrigerator to prevent degradation.

There are no recommended dietary intakes for essential fatty acids in the United States; however, studies have shown that result can be achieved from supplementing your diet with 200-400 mg of GLA and/or 400-600 ALA daily.[6,7]

Recommended dose: 2000–3000 mg of evening primrose oil and/or 1000–2000 mg of flax seed oil daily.

MSM

MSM or Methylsulfonylmethane, has grown in popularity in recent years, primarily for its alleged arthritis relieving properties. In a medical study, however, this sulfur compound was found to slightly improve hair growth by increasing the length and improving its general appearance.[8]

The sulfur in MSM is produced by the body to form keratin, the dominant protein component of hair. Some women claim they have seen an improvement in the texture of their hair, while others say they see no improvement at all. There have only been a few studies done on this supplement, and the long-term effects aren't yet known. Therefore, I do not recommend its use. It has been included in this book for informational purposes only.

SUMMARY

The effects of taking vitamins for your hair will be noticeable in 2–4 weeks. Never underestimate the power of a healthy diet! To grow healthy hair you must eat a healthy, well-rounded diet. Crash diets deprive your body of the protein and nutrition it needs which can wreck havoc on your hair. Supplement your diet with a well-rounded multi-vitamin that includes most of the recommended daily allowances of essential vitamins and minerals for your body plus extra biotin, folic acid, iron, Vitamin C, zinc and protein for your hair. Essential fatty acids provide your hair, skin and nails with the lubrication they need from the inside and are an essential part of this healthy hair regimen. But don't go overboard; taking more of than the recommended dosage will not increase hair growth and may even be harmful to your health. What your body cannot absorb or retain will be eliminated. You will be throwing your money, quite literally, down the drain.

NOTES:

10

GET MOVING!

For me, the best part about going to the salon is the shampoo. You know what I'm talking about; it's when your hairdresser leans in and gives you a vigorous shampoo that makes your scalp tingle and your toes curl. The massage feels great and it's good for you; good circulation is essential for keeping your hair healthy and radiant. Precious nutrients and oxygen flow through the blood to the scalp, where the hair is fed and subsequently grows. There are many ways to improve your circulation: scalp massages, essential oils and yoga are just a few. Yoga poses such as standing-forward-bend, downward-facing-dog and half-shoulder-stand are great ways to get your blood flowing and relieve stress. Scalp massages can help reduce tension, increase circulation, and get rid of some toxins. Essential oils smell great and can provide you with aromatherapuetic (mood enhancing) benefits as well.

SCALP MASSAGES

Scalp massages should be performed during your shampoo or on clean, dry hair (free of any gels or hairsprays.)

Tip: To allow your scalp time to heal, always wait at least a week after your relaxer before brushing or massaging.

You can massage your scalp yourself, or enlist your mate to help. To aid your massage, use massage oil.

Massage Oil

• 2 Tbls. almond, jojoba or mahabhringaraj oil

• 10–12 drops essential oil

How to Massage Your Scalp

Add a few drops of the massage oil to your fingertips. Starting at the back of your head, place all ten fingers (not nails) under your hair, on your scalp. Apply pressure in one spot by flexing and un-flexing fingers. Do this 10 times. Move toward the front and then the sides, repeating the process. Try massaging your hair before washing it to help remove dandruff using your fingers, nail-beds or knuckles. Follow with a good scalp brushing, if desired.

BRUSHING

For best results, brush your hair every other day or just before washing. Use a cushioned paddle brush or wooden massage brush designed specifically for this use. Choose a medium sized brush that fits comfortably in your hand.

Tip: Do not brush your hair with a boar or natural bristle brush because they are too damaging to relaxed hair.

How to Brush Your Scalp

Starting from the nape of your neck, brush your hair to the top of your head, bending over if necessary. Use long, slow strokes; brush up to the top, in a counter-clockwise direction. Move around your head for at least 30 strokes. Apply as much pressure as you desire.

HAIR TUGGING

It may sound strange, but hair tugging is actually a yoga pose used to increase circulation to the scalp and stimulate growth. And it feels good! Hair tugging should only be performed on dry hair. Make certain your pull from the scalp and not the ends.

How to Tug Your Hair

Grasp a handful of hair *at the scalp* and tug gently. Use firm pressure; you should feel it but it shouldn't hurt! Hold for a second or two, then tug in the hair in another direction. Hold and release. Repeat all over your head, concentrating on thin areas.

ESSENTIAL OILS

When applied to your hair and scalp, nutrients and proteins in essential oils are absorbed into the blood, giving your hair a lift. Use essential oils in a scalp massage or add them to your shampoo. Their pleasing fragrance will make your home smell inviting, and can help stimulate your senses and relieve stress.

Mahabhringaraj, also known as false daisy, is well known for its hair growth stimulating properties and is commonly used in India. Many people believe it is an excellent remedy for dandruff, premature greying, hair loss, and it may even help you sleep.

Burdock, is rich in iron, insulin and minerals. It is said to be beneficial for dandruff, eczema and psoriasis.

Cedarwood has musky scent with antiseptic properties. It may be used to treat hair loss, however, do not use on sensitive skin.

Lavender has a fresh, sweet, floral scent. It is wonderful for use on the scalp and may relieve itching, eczema, hair loss, head lice and dry scalp. Mix it with mahabhringaraj for extra special benefits.

Rosemary has a strong, camphor like scent, is colorless and is said to be an aphrodisiac. Mix it with lavender to create a magnificent massage oil. Some believe rosemary can be used to stop hair loss and may promote feelings of love and peace.

Ylang ylang, my favorite, has a seductive, sweet aroma. Aside from being an antiseptic and aphrodisiac, it may be beneficial for hair loss.

Tea tree oil has a spicy, medicinal scent. This well-known essential oil has a long list of uses. On the scalp, it helps relieve dandruff and dermatitis.

YOGA

Yoga's popularity has exploded in recent years; it seems everyone, everywhere, is doing yoga. Developed in India, yoga is an exercise with roots going back about 5,000 years; it is NOT a religion. Inverted yoga postures such as standing-forward-bend, downward-facing-dog and shoulder-stand can give your hair a boost by increasing the flow of blood to your hair follicles. I love doing yoga because it keeps me fit, yet I don't have to sweat during my workout. There is a yoga posture for everyone regardless of physical condition; to learn more about yoga, visit www.yogasite.com.

Tip: Avoid doing these poses during your period or while you are pregnant.

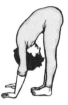

Standing-Forward-Bend

Potential benefits: Stretches the legs and spine, rests the heart and neck, improves circulation and relaxes the mind and body.

To perform this pose: Begin standing straight with your feet together. Inhale and raise your arms overhead. Exhale, bend at the hips, bring your arms forward and down until you touch the floor. **It's okay to bend your knees, especially if you're feeling stiff.** Either grasp your ankles or just let your hands dangle and breathe in and out several times. Repeat this 3–5 times. On your last bend, hold the position for 5–10 breaths. To come out of the pose, curl upward as if pulling yourself up one vertebra at a time, stacking one on top of another, and leaving the head hanging down until last.

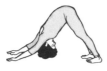

Downward-Facing-Dog

Potential benefits: Builds strength, flexibility and awareness; improves circulation; stretches the spine and hamstrings; rests the heart.

To perform this pose: Start on your hands and knees. Keep your legs about hip width apart and your arms shoulder width apart. Your middle fingers should be parallel, pointing straight ahead. Then, using your hands and feet, push with your arms and straighten your legs and push your rear end up in the air. The goal is to lengthen your spine while keeping your legs straight and your feet flat on the ground. **However, in the beginning it is okay to bend the knees a bit and to keep your heels raised.** Your weight should be evenly distributed between your hands and feet. Hold the position for a few seconds, and bit longer each day for up to 5 minutes.

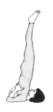

Shoulder-Stand

Potential benefits: Strengthens abdomen, stretches upper back, improves blood circulation, and induces relaxation.

To perform this pose: You probably remember doing this as a kid. Lie on your back and lift your legs up into air. Place your hands on your lower back for support, resting your elbows and lower arms on the ground. Make sure your weight is on your shoulders and mid to upper back, not your neck. Breathe deeply and hold for at the posture for at least 5–10 breaths, increasing the hold over time. To come down, slowly lower your legs, keeping them very straight (a little workout for your abdominal muscles.)

SUMMARY

Good hair and scalp care is not limited to washing and conditioning anymore. The benefits of alternative medicines and treatments are myriad and can be easily incorporated into your daily routine. They will benefit your mind, body *and* hair.

NOTES:

11

YOUR THYROID AND YOUR HAIR

What do you do if you follow the hair care regimen, eat a balanced diet, massage your scalp and your hair continues to shed? It may be diffuse hair loss attributed to a thyroid disorder. The thyroid is a small, butterfly shaped gland located in the base of the throat. It secretes hormones that regulate your metabolism, the rate at which cells function, including hair cells. When your thyroid produces too many or too few hormones, problems will result. Thyroid disease affects 1 in every 10 people and is considered a genetic disease. Many times, people ignore their symptoms, thinking they are tolerable or even acceptable because they are similar to stress. Indications of thyroid disease include depression, fatigue, irritability and unexplained weight loss or gain, which can be confused with depression or even PMS. It is for this reason so many people go undiagnosed. Thyroid disease primarily affects women between the ages of 18–35, but can affect anyone. Even a slight hormone imbalance can have a major effect on your body and your hair. Take the thyroid assessment quiz below to see if you are at risk.

THYROID RISK ASSESSMENT

1. Does anyone in your family have thyroid disease?

2. Have you had any unexplained weight loss or gain (more than 10 pounds) in the past six months?

3. Take your pulse for ten seconds. Multiply the number by six. Is the result greater than 100 or less than 60?

4. Have you been shedding (whole hair, contains bulb) more than 100 hairs a day?

5. Has you hair texture changed in the last six months?

6. Are you frequently fatigued?

7. Are you depressed?

8. Are you sensitive to hot or cold temperatures?

9. Are you having trouble sleeping?

10. Do your hands tremble?

If you answered yes to more than three of the questions above, talk with your doctor.

There are several different kinds of thyroid disease, primarily **hypothyroidism** (too little) and **hyperthyroidism** (too much).

An overactive thyroid (hyperthyroidism) affects your hair in two ways. The hair cells are created so quickly that they are not complete, resulting in thin, soft hair that will not hold a curl. Second, thyroid hormones may speed the body up so much that the body's energy must be diverted from the hair follicles, shutting them down just to keep up with demand. This causes your hair to go into the telogen (resting) phase early, resulting in hair loss.

Symptoms of Hyperthyroidism	Symptoms of Hypothyroidism
Trembling hands	Sluggish pulse
Heart rate over 100	Pulse rate under 60
Racing pulse	Weight gain
Weight loss	Depression
Increased appetite	Decreased appetite
Hair loss	Hair loss
Dry skin and hair	Dry, coarse skin and hair
Soft hair that won't hold a curl	Constipation
Diarrhea	Intolerance to cold (can't get warm)
Intolerance to heat	"Bug" eyes
Muscle weakness	Swollen neck
Excessive sweating	Fatigue
Dry eyes	Muscle cramps
Fatigue	Mood swings
Irritability	
Mood swings	
Insomnia	
Fine, brittle hair	

In hypothyroidism, the effects are similar. The body's energy is so depleted that it shuts down "unnecessary'" activity (including hair follicles) to conserve energy. The hair that does grow grows at such a slow, exaggerated rate that the hairs texture becomes dry and coarse.

Fortunately, most thyroid disease is easily treatable with medication, usually for life. Unfortunately, medications such as levoxythroin and Synthroid® may cause hair loss as well (read the prescription insert).

So what should you do if you take thyroid medication?

1. **Get your thyroid levels under control.** Internal and external factors can cause the body's need for thyroid hormone to fluctuate. If you experience any of the symptoms for hyperthyroidism, including persistent hair loss, your dosage may be too high or too low. Talk with your doctor if you aren't feeling well or if your symptoms return.

2. **Consider T3.** Synthetic thyroid hormones are primarily T4 (thyroxine). However, some patients do better on a combination of T4 and T3 (triiodothyronine). Ask your doctor if supplementing with T3 could be right for you.

3. **Take 2000–3000 mg evening primrose oil daily.** Evening primrose oil is rich is GLA, which the body converts to hormones called prostaglandins. Prostaglandins act similar to thyroid hormones and supplementation of GLA can help ease your symptoms.

4. **Get a haircut.** If your hair loss is severe, get a haircut, and keep it trimmed to stay at that length. Your hair will fill out as new hair grows in and catches up with the older hair. Try thickening shampoos like Thicker, Fuller Hair, to swell hair strands and make your mane look fuller.

5. **Learn to deal with stress.** The body's need for thyroid hormone can be affected by stress. Learn stress management techniques including deep breathing, meditation and prayer.

6. **Eat a well balanced, healthy diet.** Avoid dieting and therefore stressing your body until your thyroid hormone levels are under control. As your levels stabilize, your metabolism will speed up, and you will lose weight.

7. **Last, take great care of your hair** by following the healthy hair regimen in this book.

NOTES:

_____

_____

_____

_____

_____

_____

_____

_____

_____

_____

_____

_____

_____

12

NO-HEAT STYLE GUIDE

In this chapter, you will find step-by-step instructions for creating five healthy hair styles. Rotate them for variety and use your imagination to make each style your own! All of these styles can be achieved without heat and will look great for a few days. Whatever your personal style or hair length, these hair styles will provide you with plenty of options without sacrificing style. Get creative!

For more information and photos of these styles and more, visit http:// www.hbhonline.com.

THE WRAP

The **wrap** is a style in which your hair is wrapped in a circular motion around your head while wet. Once dry, your hair should be smooth and straight. I remember when the wrap first came out, in 1990. I hated it! It was so boring, so...*flat* (after the big haired eighties.) I had no idea that this style would change my hair forever. My hair was really short back then, it ended about an inch above my ears. I wrapped my hair consistently until the time I moved to Atlanta, when my hair was almost to my shoulders.

Supplies You Will Need

• 1:4 setting lotion mixture

• Fine tooth comb

• Wide tooth comb

• Leave-in conditioner

• Shine detangler

• Sanek® paper (or toilet paper)

• Hair oil or oil sheen

Step One — Prepare Your Hair

Wash, condition and gently towel blot your hair. Then, add a little leave-in conditioner, a good dollop of gloss and a few drops of oil. Make sure all of the products are distributed evenly.

Step Two — Set

Saturate your hair with your 1:4 setting lotion mixture. Don't soak your hair; however, make sure it is completely covered because it will be smoothed on your head and you need the setting lotion to hold it in place while it dries.

Detangle your hair using the wide tooth comb. Start combing from the top of your hair down in all directions. After the tangles are removed, comb through your hair in the same manner with a fine tooth comb a few times to smooth it out.

Step Three — Wrap

Using your fine tooth comb, start at the top of your head. With short strokes, gently swirl a 1½ inch wide section of your hair in a clockwise (or counter-clockwise) direction. Gather more hair as you go along, combing with one hand and then smoothing the wrapped hair down with the other. You may need to press the comb down flat to get the hair smooth.

Continue to swirl your hair slowly around your ears, across the forehead and behind the other ear.

A good wrap is truly an art form and takes a lot of practice, but you will be a pro in no time. Don't get discouraged if yours isn't completely smooth. If it's a mess, comb your hair down gently using the wide tooth comb and try again. Take your time. If you can't get it quite right, that's ok; dry it anyway. Just do the best you can and you'll be fine.

To hold the wrap in place while it dries, use Sanek® (stretchy tissue paper) or toilet paper. Wrap the paper around your head on top of the hair in the same direction as your wrap. Be careful not to mess up your handiwork! Use the paper to help press your wrap smooth. Overlap the ends of the paper in front of your head, above your forehead and secure it. Glue them together with a few squirts of setting lotion.

Step Four — Dry

Dry your wrap overnight, or under a warm dryer. If you will be using a dryer plan on at least 45 minutes for short hair to 90 minutes for long hair. When drying your hair overnight sit under the dryer first for at least 5–10 minutes to remove excess moisture.

Then, use a satin do-rag instead of tissue paper to hold your hair in place. The satin won't absorb water from your hair and will allow it to breathe (dry). Cotton will retain moisture.

Step Five — Style and Maintain

After your hair is dry (you can check by gently combing your fingers through) add a few drops of oil to your palms and smooth them on your hair to "break" the wrap (it will be a little crispy). Using your wide tooth comb, comb in the direction of the wrap first, then down. Part your hair and go!

To keep your wrap fresh, wrap it back up at night with your paddle brush. Add a few drops of oil each night around your hair-line and on your ends. Tie it up tight with a do-rag or silk scarf.

SPLIT-WRAP

As your hair grows or if you are having trouble getting a good wrap, try a **split-wrap.** In a split-wrap the top half of your hair is set on a roller and the rest is wrapped. This helps reduce drying time and will add body and bounce to your style. Because you will be using jumbo rollers (as large as your hair length will allow) the curls will be loose and sexy. When I wear my hair down, this is my favorite way to style my hair. I do this at night and let it dry overnight.

Additional Supplies Needed

- 3 or 4 jumbo rollers (as large as your hair will allow, 1 or 1½ inches)

- Roller clips or pins

Step One — Prepare Your Hair

Wash and condition your hair, then add your leave-ins: leave-in conditioner, oil and gloss.

Step Two — Set

Lightly spray your 1:4 setting lotion mixture all over your hair. You will be brushing your curls out, so they should be loose and bouncy, not hard and crispy. Detangle your hair first using the wide tooth comb. Start combing from the top of your hair; combing the front part of your hair down toward your face, the sides toward your ears and the back of your hair down towards the floor. Once all the tangles are removed, comb through your hair in the same manner with a fine tooth comb a few times to smooth it out.

Step Three — Roll

Divide a large square section of your hair at the top of your head. You will be setting this section on rollers.

To roll, separate a small 1 by 2 inch piece of your hair, then comb the section up until smooth. Place a large roller behind the section of hair (you will roll towards the back of your head) and smooth the ends over. Slowly roll the roller down toward your head until it rests on your head, then secure. Repeat this process in the sections directly adjacent to the roller. Depending on the length of your hair, you will have 4–5 rollers, one in the center, and one in front, one in the back and two on each side.

Step Four — Wrap

Using the fine tooth comb, start at the back of your head, just under the rollers. Being careful not to disturb your rollers, gently swirl a 1½ inch section of the hair in a clockwise (or counter-clockwise) direction. Gather more hair as you go along, pressing the comb down flat to keep your hair smooth until you reach your ears. Swirl your hair up and around your ears, across your forehead and behind your other ear. Hold your wrap in place with Sanek® tissue paper or toilet paper and cover the rollers with a hair net.

Step Four — Dry

Dry either under the dryer or air-dry. If you are going to sleep, cover your curls with a hair net then secure the wrapped portion with a long satin scarf. If you cover the hair net with the scarf your style is guaranteed to stay in place.

Step Five — Style and Maintain

After your hair is dry, remove the rollers first, then add a few drops of oil to your entire head. Using a paddle brush or wide tooth comb, brush the curls and wrapped hair together, then down. If your hair is too curly on top, brush all of your hair into a wrap, leave it in for a few minutes, then brush it down. Part your hair and style as desired.

To keep your split-wrap fresh, wrap it back up at night using your paddle brush. You can add a few rollers if you like, as well as a few drops of oil around your hairline and on your ends.

THE UP-DO

The up-do is an extremely versatile style. Wear it with a long, straight bang or pile of spiral curls. It's great to wear to the office, the club or for everyday.

Supplies You Will Need

• 1:1 Setting lotion mixture

• Protein gel

• Ponytail holder

• Bobby pins

• Hair pins

• Fine tooth comb

• Wide tooth comb

• Rollers

• Roller clips or pins

• Hair oil

• Shine Gloss

Step One — Prepare Your Hair

Wash, condition and gently towel blot your hair. Add leave-in conditioner and saturate it with the setting lotion mixture. Some gloss will help to detangle and a few drops of oil will add sheen to your style.

Step Two — Divide

Have a good idea of what you want your up-do to look like. The back of your hair will be swept up, leaving the bangs free to style as you wish. Divide your hair into two sections; one for your bang and the other for the knot. Depending on how you want your bang to look, the front section of your hair will be divided into a shape, and the rest will be gathered together to make the roll.

A. **Square.** If you want spiral curls in front, section a wide, square bang from your outer eyebrow to the top all the way back to the center top of your head.

B. **Rectangle.** For an elegant twist, eliminate the bang and sweep your hair to the side like you would a wrap. Section from the outer eyebrows back a few inches and across.

C. **Triangle.** Another option is a long bang that can be worn straight or with a curl. Section diagonally from the outer eyebrows back to the center most part of your head to form a triangular shape.

Divide, then detangle your hair, combing it into the two sections.

Step Three — Set

Slick the back section of your hair back with your fine tooth comb to smooth it out. Then, add a small amount of protein gel to keep the hair on the sides in place (optional). Gather this section of your hair into a ponytail, in the center of the back of your head. Set the hair of your ponytail onto one or more jumbo rollers and secure.

Next, set or wrap the front bang depending on your style.

A. Square. See the section on roller sets for help how to achieve spiral or large curls.

B. Rectangle. Apply protein gel to your hair before wrapping it. Using short strokes, comb your hair flat and smooth. Sweep it low across your forehead and behind the opposite ear.

C. Triangle. Divide this section of your hair in two and set each section on a jumbo roller.

Step Four — Dry

Dry under a warm dryer for 45–60 minutes.

Step Five — Style and Maintain

Once your hair is dry, remove your ponytail first. Add a few drops of oil to your palms and scrunch it on the back section of your hair. Using a paddle brush or wide tooth comb, brush your hair up and to one side, then secure it with bobby pins. Your hair should be sticking up on one side.

Fold your hair over the bobby pin so it doesn't show and secure it with a hair pin. Then, slowly roll and tuck the rest of your hair into a roll securing it with hair pins. Tuck more and more hair into the roll until you get to the top. Smooth the top of your roll and secure. Remove the rollers from the front of your hair. Again, add a small amount of oil to your hands and scrunch on the curls. Then, simply style them as desired.

To maintain this style, cover your hair with a satin bonnet at night. Use rollers if necessary to tighten loose curls.

ROLLER SET

The roller set is the mainstay of the healthy hair regimen. It's not your grandmother's roller set! Rollers can be used to make tight, spiral curls, or giant sexy waves. Roller sets are long-lasting and when done properly, make your hair dry straighter. They last well and can be worn in any number or styles. Roller sets take practice, but you can master them. With practice it will become second nature to you and you will find yourself wondering why you ever used a curling iron.

You will need to purchase 12–36 rollers, depending on your hair length and the size of the roller. I recommend using magnetic rollers without the snap-on cover as the covers leave dents. However, snap-on rollers are good to use at night and to refresh curls. Never use sponge or cloth rollers.

Supplies You Will Need

- Magnetic rollers

    — **For short hair:** purchase 12 to 24 $\frac{1}{4}$- to $\frac{1}{2}$-inch rollers

    — **For medium length hair:** purchase 18 to 24 $\frac{1}{2}$- or 1-inch rollers.

    — **For long hair:** purchase 24 1-inch rollers, 24 to 36 $\frac{1}{4}$- or $\frac{1}{2}$-inch rollers or 18 to 24 1$\frac{1}{2}$-inch rollers.

- 36 hair clips

- Bobby pins

- Setting lotion mixture (1:1 for hard sets or spiral curls; 1:4 for loose sets)

- Wide tooth comb

• Fine tooth comb

• Gloss

• Hair oil or sheen

• Leave-in conditioner

Step One — Prepare Your Hair

Washing, conditioning and adding your leave-in styling aids (leave-in conditioner, oil and gloss) will prepare your hair for this style.

Step Two — Set

Using your fine tooth comb, divide a large square section of your hair from your outer eyebrow back to the top of your hair and across. Clip the other hair back and out of the way. Then, spritz this section with your preferred setting lotion mixture.

Within this section, at the top of your head, separate a 1-inch by 2-inch wide piece of hair. Comb it upward until smooth. Place the roller behind your hair and smooth the end over the middle of the roller. Hold your finger over the hair on the roller and then roll the roller down towards your head.

Keeping a good grip, gently pull the roller up to remove any slack, and then secure the roller to your head (using a clip.) Repeat throughout your entire head. Depending on the length of your hair, you will have 3–5 sections: one on top, one on each side and two for the back of your hair.

For spiral curls, spritz your hair with a stronger solution of setting lotion first, 1:1 parts. Your curls will dry crispy. To set, repeat the process above but use less hair on each roller (about a 1 by 1 inch piece.) Comb your hair up until smooth and then smooth the ends of your hair over the *bottom end* of the roller. Turn the roller vertical and then slowly roll the roller down, wrapping your hair higher up on the roller in a corkscrew motion. Before securing the roller, gently pull the roller tight, then secure with a clip. Repeat this process, covering your whole head.

Step Four — Dry

Dry your roller set under the dryer as air-drying may take several hours. Plan on at least 45 minutes for short hair to 60 minutes or longer for long hair. Roller sets do not dry well overnight.

Step Five — Style and Maintain

Once your hair is dry (you can check by removing one or two rollers) remove all of the rollers. You may want to sit under the dryer for an additional minute or two after you do so, just to make sure your scalp is completely dry. Add a few drops of oil to hand and 'scrunch' it on your hair but don't break your curls. Then, style as desired, brushing your curls smooth, or separating them with your fingers.

To keep your curls fresh, cover them at night with a satin sleep cap, adding a few rollers if needed. Or, when your curls start to fall, use your paddle brush to brush them into a wrap and wrap with a scarf. Wrapping will remove the rest of the curl, leaving your hair straight but full of bounce. Or pin up the back of your hair for an elegant up-do.

BRAID-OUT

A braid-out is an easy, textured hair style that is great to wear during the summer or while on vacation. Your hair is braided or twisted while wet and then dried, producing long-lasting waves and crimps. Try air-drying your braid-out overnight.

Supplies You Will Need

• Wide tooth comb

• Shine detangler

• Hair oil

• Setting lotion mixture

• Rollers (optional)

• Roller clips or pins

Step One — Prepare Your Hair

Wash and condition your hair, then prepare it with leave-in conditioner, gloss and oil.

Step Two — Set

Saturate your hair with your 1:1 setting lotion mixture and detangle. Don't use gel.

Step Three — Set

A. Cornrows. You will be dividing your hair in to 3–5 sections, depending on the length of your hair, and the size of the waves you prefer. Use three sections for loose waves (one on each side and one down the middle) and five for kinky waves.

NOTE: Your part should not be straight — a crooked part will work better. If your parts are too deep, your hair will stay separated when it's dry.

Starting with the side section, lightly divide your hair from front to back. Clip the rest of your hair away from the section. Beginning at the front, braid your hair in a French braid or cornrow, taking in more hair as you go along. When you reach the end, secure the end of the braid with a clip or set it on a jumbo roller. Repeat this process with the other sections.

B. Individual Braids. For wild crimps, repeat the process from above, but braid your hair into individual braids instead of cornrows.

C. Twists. Twists are done a little differently. You will be using smaller sections (between 1–2 inches) depending on your style. If you wear a part, create it first then work around it. Starting in the back, section a square shaped section of your hair. Separate it in two, then twist it together tightly from the scalp up. For more texture, twist it around in a "knot" or simply secure the end with a bobby pin. Repeat this process for your entire head.

Step Four — Dry

Braid-outs can take longer to dry than sets or wraps. Plan on at least 60 minutes under the dryer, which is why I recommend letting your braid-out dry overnight. When doing this, make sure your ends are covered with a satin sleep cap or hairnet.

Step Five — Style and Maintain

Once your hair is dry and you have taken out your braids, add a few drops of oil and gloss to your hair. Fluff your style with your fingers or use a wide tooth comb. You can add barrettes, a headband or pull your hair into ponytail on top of your head. Braid-outs can feel dry or look frizzy, so be sure to use your hair oil and gloss daily. At night, cover your style with a sleep cap and re-braid or twist sections that are losing their shape. Spritz them lightly with water and let them dry overnight.

NOTES:

APPENDIX A:
TEST ANSWERS

Answers to the Scalp Health Assessment from Page 15:

1. A. 1..........B. 0..............C. 2

2. A. 1..........B. 3

3. A. 3..........B. 1..............C. 6

4. A. 3..........B. 0

5. A. 1..........B. 0

6. A. 3..........B. 0

7. A. 3..........B. 0

8. A. 6..........B. 0

Scoring

0–6 points

Your symptoms indicate that you may have dermatitis. Turn to page 19 for more information.

7–14 points

Your symptoms indicate that you may have dandruff. Turn to page 16 for more information.

15 + points

Your symptoms indicate that you may have scalp psoriasis. Turn to page 19 for more information.

Answers to the Hair Type Test from Page 21:

1. A. 0..........B. 2 ✗
2. A. 0..........B. 2
3. A. 2✗.........B. 0
4. A. 0..........B. 2
5. A. 2..........B. 0
6. A. 1..........B. 0
7. A. 2..........B. 0
8. A. 2✗.........B. 0
9. A. 0..........B. 1
10. A. 0..........B. 1...............C. 2   D. 4
11. A. 2..........B. 0...............C. 1

Scoring

0–8 points
Your hair is healthy. Turn to page 23 for your hair care regimen.

10–18 points
Your hair is stressed or dry. Turn to page 25 for your hair care regimen.

19+ points
Your hair is damaged. Turn to page 27 for your hair care regimen.

HEALTHY HAIR DO'S & DON'TS

Healthy Hair Do's

- Do eat a healthy diet

- Do stimulate your scalp regularly

- Do limit the use of heat on your hair

- Do use a wide tooth comb for styling

- Do protect your hair from the sun with sunscreen or by wearing a hat

- Do reduce stress whenever possible

- Do use quality products

- Do use satin pillowcases

- Do treat scalp disorders

- Do protect your hair at night

- Do wear your hair up often

- Do use the same brand of relaxer consistently

- Do stick with the same type of relaxer (lye, no lye)

- Do get a hair trim 2–3 times a year

- Do oil your ends and hairline daily

- Do exfoliate your scalp during shampoo

- Do supplement your diet with vitamins, minerals and essential fatty acids

- Do use cushioned paddle brushes to brush your hair

- Do use semi-permanent (Level 1, deposit only) hair color

- Do get highlights instead of using permanent hair color

- Do get perms regularly, every 7–9 weeks

- Do deep condition (with heat) once or twice a week

- Do rub medicated shampoos into the scalp and not just your hair

- Do massage your scalp

- Do wash your hair twice a week or every four days to keep your scalp clean

- Do use hair pins with coated ends

- Do use drawstring ponytails or clip on hair

- Do use hot oil treatments regularly to relieve dandruff

- Do use Tea Tree oil on your scalp to relieve itching

- Do get large braids or wear cornrows frequently

- Do take a Break at least once a year

Healthy Hair Don'ts

- Don't go on crash diets

- Don't avoid hair trims but...

- Don't squander hair growth by getting hair trims too frequently (more than 2–3 times a year)

- Don't use heat regularly

- Don't comb your hair with a fine tooth comb

- Don't use natural or boar bristle brushes

- Don't switch back and forth between relaxer brands

- Don't use a lye perm after a no-lye perm

- Don't use permanent hair color

- Don't use pin-on hair (only clip-on or drawstring)

- Don't wait longer than 10 weeks to get a perm.

- Don't use hair sprays or styling gels (only protein gel or pomade)

- Don't use rubber bands on your hair

- Don't use weave glue

- Don't use hair pins without coated ends

- Don't hot curl wet hair or use hair spray when hot curling your hair

- Don't scratch your dandruff

- Don't blow-dry hair when it's wet (air-dry first)

- Don't get micro-braids

- Don't go 2 weeks without washing your hair (unless you have braids)

- Don't use commercial braid sprays

- Don't scratch excessively

- Don't scratch your scalp with a pencil or bobby pins

- Don't put weave glue directly on your scalp

- Don't pick at scabs or scales

- Don't get a perm on an unhealthy scalp

- Don't put Seabreeze® in your hair prior to a perm

- Don't grease your scalp with petroleum-based products

FOOTNOTES

1 From page 19:
http://www3.gov.ab.ca/hre/whs/publications/pdf/ch001.pdf

2 From page 62:
http://www.cfsan.fda.gov/~dms/fdahdye.html

3 From page 81:
Morse P, Horrobin D, Manku M. *Meta-analysis of Placebo-controlled Studies of the Efficacy of Evening Primrose Oil (Epogam in the Treatment of Atopic Eczema.*

4 From page 81:
Jakubowica D. *The Significance Of Prostaglandins In The Pre-Menstrual Syndrome. In: Taylor R, Ed. Premenstrual Syndrome. London: Medical New-Tribune, 1983, p.16.*

5 From page 81:
relationship Between Plasma Essential Fatty Acid Changes and Clinical Response. British Journal of Dermatology, 1989; 121:75–90.

6 From page 82:
Horrobin K. *Calcium Metabolism, Osteoporosis and Essential Fatty Acids: A Review.* Progress in Lipid Research, 1997; 36(2–3):131–151

7 From page 82:
Horrobin D. *Review of Contemporary Pharmacotherapy,* 1990; 1:1–45.

8 From page 82:
Lawrence, Ronald M. M.D., PhD *The Effectiveness of the Use of Oral LIGNISULmsm (Methylsulfonylmethane) Supplementation on Hair & Nail Health* Council for Natural Nutrition 2/2/01.

REFERENCES

Budd, Martin, MD. *Why Am I So Tired? Is Your Thyroid Making You Ill?* Thorsons, Hammersmith, London. 2000

Janssen, Mary Beth. *Naturally Healthy Hair : Herbal Treatments And Daily Care For Fabulous Hair.* Story Books, Pownel, VT 1999

Larger, Stephen E., Scheer, James F., *Solved: The Riddle of Illness, Your Amazing Thyroid,* 3rd Edition. Keats Publishing, 2000

Morse, Nancy L. *Evening Primrose Oil.* Alive Books, 2002

Pressman, Alan H. *The Complete Idiot's Guide to Vitamins and Minerals.* Alpha Books, New York, NY 1997.

Rosenthal, M. Sara. *the Thyroid Sourcebook for Women,* Lowell House, Lincolnwood, IL 1999

Springhouse Corporation. *Everything you Need to Know about Medical Treatments,* Springhouse Corporation, 1996

www.yogasite.com

BIBLIOGRAPHY

Budd, Martin, MD. *Why Am I So Tired? Is Your Thyroid Making You Ill?* Thorsons, Hammersmith, London. 2000

Edelson, Gary W. MD. *Your Thyroid Gland; A Guide for Thyroid Patients,* 3rd Edition. Associated Endocrinologists, 1993

Freid, John J, Petska, Sharon. *The American Druggist's Comprehensive Family Guide to Prescriptions, Pills and Drugs,* 1st Edition. Hearst Books, New York, NY 1995

Griffith, H. Winter. *Healing Herbs; The Essential Guide,* Fisher Books, Phoenix, AZ. 2000

___ *Comprehensive Guide to Prescription and Non-Prescription Drugs,* 1st Edition. Penguin Publishing, New York NY, 2001

Janssen, Mary Beth. *Naturally Healthy Hair: Herbal Treatments and Daily Care for Fabulous Hair.* Story Books, Pownel, VT 1999

Larger, Stephen E.; Scheer, James F. Solved: *The Riddle of Illness, Your Amazing Thyroid,* 3rd Edition. Keats Publishing, 2000

The Medical Advisor: The Complete Guide to Alternative & Conventional Treatments / By the Editors of Time-Life Books, 2nd Edition. Time Life Books, 2000

Milady's Standard Textbook Of Cosmetology, Milady Publishing Company. 2000

Morse, Nancy L. *Evening Primrose Oil.* Alive Books, 2002

Peirce, Andrea. *The American Pharmaceutical Association Practical Guide to Natural Medicines,* 1st Edition. The Stonesong Press Inc., 1999

Perricone, Nicholas, MD. *The Wrinkle Cure; Unlock the Power of Cosmecueticals for Supple, Youthful Skin,* Rodale Inc, 2000

Physician's Desk Reference Medical Dictionary, 1st Edition, Medical Economics, Montral, NJ 1995.

Physician's Desk Reference for Non-Prescription Drugs and Dietary Supplements, Medical Economics, Montral NJ, 1995

Physician's Desk Reference for Herbal Medicines, Medical Economics, Montral NJ, 1995

www.omeganutrition.com

Pressman, Alan H. *The Complete Idiot's Guide to Vitamins and Minerals,* Alpha Books, New York, NY 1997.

Prevention's Healing With Vitamins, Rodale Press, 1996

Rosenthal, M. Sara. *The Thyroid Sourcebook for Women,* Lowell House, Lincolnwood, IL 1999

Springhouse Corporation. *Everything You Need to Know About Medical Treatments.* Springhouse Corporation, 1996

Ternus, Maureen. *The Everything Vitamins, Minerals and Nutritional Supplements Book.* 1st Edition. 2001

Winter, Ruth. *A Consumer's Dictionary of Cosmetic Ingredients,* 4th edition. Random House, New York, NY. 1994

www.yogasite.com

GLOSSARY

Almond oil—A light, odorless oil that is rich in protein, vitamins and minerals.

Alpha lineolenic acid (ALA)—An essential fatty acid that belongs to the Omega 3 family that may help some skin disorders.

Amino acids—Also known as "the building blocks of protein" they can penetrate the cuticle layer. When added to hair products they impart sheen, moisture and improve the hair's general condition.

Ammonium laureth sulfate—Cleansing agent used to break up oils and soils so they can be removed from hair and skin.

Ammonium lauryl sulfate—A mild surfactant widely used at acidic (mild) pH values.

Anagen—Phase in which hair is growing.

Biotin—A naturally occurring vitamin H. May have a positive effect on hair growth when taken internally.

Bulb—A white sheath that protects the papilla.

Burdock—An essential oil rich in iron and minerals that may be beneficial for dandruff, eczema and psoriasis.

Catagen—Resting phase for the hair follicle during which hair is preparing itself for removal.

Cedarwood—Has antiseptic properties. May be beneficial for hair loss.

Consultation—Appointment with a hairdresser during which s/he will determine the health of your hair and scalp.

Cortex—Middle layer of the hair shaft where structural and color changes take place.

Cuticle—Outer layer of the hair shaft that protects the cortex. Consists of several layers of dead keratin cells or scales.

Cyclomethicone—A silicone derivative that adds luster and sheen and emollients benefits. Can be used as a carrier for other ingredients.

Dandruff—Skin condition that is characterized by white flakes and itching.

Dermatitis—Skin condition that does not respond to moisture.

Dermis—Lower layer of the scalp consisting of sebaceous glands, hair follicles, nerve endings and blood vessels.

Dimethicone—A silicone derivative. Adds luster and sheen.

Drawstring ponytail—An add-on hair piece in which a ponytail is inserted, then secured by pulling the drawstring closed.

Epidermis—Outer layer of the skin.

Essential fatty acids—Macronutrients required by the body. Essential fatty acids include Omega 3 (3 carbon), omega 6 (6 carbon) and omega 9 (9 carbon).

Essential oils—Used for fragrance, antiseptics, germicides and natural moisturizers. Derived from natural plant oil.

Evening primrose oil—Rich in gamma linoliec acid (GLA).

Finishing agents—Substances added to cosmetic products to soften and smooth the cuticle layer.

Flax seed oil—An excellent source of alpha lineolenic acid (ALA).

Gamma linoliec acid (GLA)—An essential fatty acid belonging to the Omega 6 family.

Glycerin—General humectant and moisturizer.

Guanidine hydroxide—A mix of calcium hydroxide and guanidine carbonate used in hair straighteners.

Hair follicle—Houses the hair root.

Humectants—Substances which are added to cosmetic products to hold and retain moisture.

Hydrolysis—A process in which substances are turned partly into water.

Hydrolyzed proteins—Proteins subject to hydrolysis. Examples include animal, milk, keratin, collagen, wheat, human placenta and human hair protein.

Hyperthyroidism—A condition in which the thyroid gland produces excess hormones.

Hypothyroid—A condition in which the thyroid gland produces too few hormones to meet the body's needs.

Jojoba oil—Derived from the seed of the jojoba shrub. Excellent softening and moisturizing qualities; lightweight, easily absorbed and contains nutrients for the skin.

Keratin—Protein obtained from animals.

Keratin amino acids—A mixture of amino acids from the hydrolysis (see) of keratin.

Lavender—An essential oil that has a sweet, floral scent and may help relieve itching, eczema, hair loss and dry scalp.

Lye—See sodium hydroxide.

Mahabhringaraj—Also known as false daisy. Well known hair oil used in India.

Medulla—Inner core of the hair shaft that gives the hair stiffness and strength. May be absent or fragmented.

Melanin—Cells within the cortex that gives the hair its color.

Methylsulfonylmethane—Also known as MSM. A naturally occurring source of sulfur found in all living organisms and is present in our body fluids and tissues.

Mineral oil—Finishing agent. A mixture of refined liquid hydrocarbons derived from petroleum.

Minoxidil—Works as a hair growth stimulant for some.

Olive oil—Obtained by pressing olives and is rich in protein, vitamins and minerals. Has a heavier weight than other oils and a strong aroma. Available in extra–virgin (oil from first pressing of olives) and virgin (last pressing) varieties.

Panthenol—Member of the Vitamin B complex family; used as a hair thickener and conditioning agent. During oxidation it is converted to Vitamin B-5 (pantheonic acid). Derivations include ethyl panthenol. Improves the condition of damaged hair and gives the hair gloss.

Papilla—Part of the hair root where hair cells are created.

Perm cycle—Amount of time between perms, preferably 7–9 weeks.

Petroleum—Purified mixture of semi-solid hydrocarbons the hair is unable to absorb.

pH—Potential hydrogen.

Pityriasis capitis simplex—Dandruff.

Pityrosporum ovale—Dandruff-causing fungus.

Pityriasis steatoides—Contagious type of dandruff.

Propylene glycol—Mixture of propylene glycol and coconut fatty acids. An excellent humectant and also aids in removing product build-up from hair.

Psoriasis—Skin condition in which the rate of cell growth is accelerated and results in thick scales.

Root—hair follicle.

Rosemary—Has a strong, camphor like scent, is colorless and may help hair loss.

Sebum—Secreted by the sebaceous glands. Nourishes the hair and scalp.

Shaft—Hair that grows above the skin. Consists of the cuticle, cortex and medulla.

Shea butter—Natural fat obtained from the fruit of the Karite tree. Used as a replacement for lanolin.

Sodium hydroxide—Lye. Alkaline, caustic chemical used in hair straighteners and cuticle removers.

Sodium laureth sulfate—Derivative of polyethylene glycol and lauryl alcohol. Milder than sodium lauryl sulfate and may be used in conjunction with other surfactants.

Sodium lauryl sulfate—Derivative of polyethylene glycol and lauryl alcohol. Recommended for use in conjunction with other surfactants.

Sorbitol—Moisturizing agent and lubricant. Has similar properties to glycerin but is more compatible with hair.

Tea tree oil—Antiseptic derived from the Australian melaleuca alternafolia plant.

Telogen—Phase during which a new hair strand is created.

Telogen effluvium—Entering the telogen phase prematurely, usually due to an illness or medication.

Thyroxine—Also known as T4. Hormone secreted by the thyroid. Thyroid hormones are 93% thyroxine.

Triiodothyronine—Also known as T3. Hormone secreted by the thyroid that accounts for about 7% of the hormones secreted.

Wheat germ oil—Contains antioxidants and vitamins A, B, C, D and E.

Wrap—A hairstyle in which the hair is wrapped in a circular motion around the head.

Ylang ylang—Has a seductive, sweet aroma. May be beneficial for hair loss.

INDEX

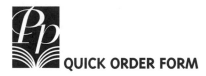

QUICK ORDER FORM

Fax Orders: Fax to (325) 202-8156. Send this form.

Telephone Orders: Call (877) 723-6110. Have your credit card ready.

Email orders: *sales@panaceapublishing.com.*

Postal Orders: Panacea Publishing, Order Dept., PO BOX 395, Bloomfield Hills, MI 48303-0395, USA. Telephone: (877) 723-6110

■ **Please send the following:**

☐ Healthy Black Hair ☐ Healthy Black Hair Starter Kit

☐ Healthy Black Hair for Teens ☐ Healthy Black Hair Diary

■ **Please send more FREE information on:**

☐ Other Books ☐ Volume Sales ☐ Seminars ☐ Authors

Name: _____

Address: _____

City/State/Zip: _____

Sales Tax: Please add 6% for products shipped to Michigan addresses.

Shipping by air:
US: $4 for the first book and add $2.00 for each additional product.
International: $9 for the first book; $5 for each additional (estimate.)

Payment:

☐ Check   ☐ Credit Card (circle one): Visa   MC   AMEX   Discover

Card No. _____

Name on Card: _____

Exp. Date: _____/_____

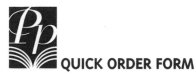

QUICK ORDER FORM

Fax Orders: Fax to (325) 202-8156. Send this form.

Telephone Orders: Call (877) 723-6110. Have your credit card ready.

Email orders: *sales@panaceapublishing.com.*

Postal Orders: Panacea Publishing, Order Dept., PO BOX 395, Bloomfield Hills, MI 48303-0395, USA. Telephone: (877) 723-6110

■ **Please send the following:**

❑ Healthy Black Hair   ❑ Healthy Black Hair Starter Kit

❑ Healthy Black Hair for Teens   ❑ Healthy Black Hair Diary

■ **Please send more FREE information on:**

❑ Other Books   ❑ Volume Sales   ❑ Seminars   ❑ Authors

Name: _____

Address: ___ _____

City/State/Zip: _____

Sales Tax: Please add 6% for products shipped to Michigan addresses.

Shipping by air:
US: $4 for the first book and add $2.00 for each additional product.
International: $9 for the first book; $5 for each additional (estimate.)

Payment:

❑ Check   ❑ Credit Card (circle one): Visa   MC   AMEX   Discover

Card No. _____

Name on Card: _____

Exp. Date: _____/_____